The
Vegan Guide
To
New York City

RYNN BERRY & CHRIS A. SUZUKI

With Barry Litsky, J.D.

Published by

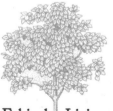

Ethical | Living

This book is dedicated to FM Esfandiary, Napoleao Nelson Salgado-Santos, and to all people who respect animals enough not to eat them or consume their byproducts.

•

Eighteenth edition, 2012

ISBN 13: 978-0-9788132—5-3
ISBN 10: 0-9788132 5-1

Library of Congress Number 2001-135857

This book is printed on durable, acid-free paper.

Published in the United States by Ethical Living
P O Box 8174
JAF Station
New York, NY 10116

Cover design and title page design by Donna Hughes; Dr. Chris Abreu-Suzuki, and Vrinda Berasi. Cover drawing by Sarah Caplan. Copyright © by Rynn Berry and Chris Abreu-Suzuki.

Our thanks to Carolyn Handel, Diane Brandt, and J.C. Oliveira.

HanGawi Restaurant

a vegetarian shrine in another space and time

**Voted top vegetarian restaurant in NYC
- Zagat Survey 2010**

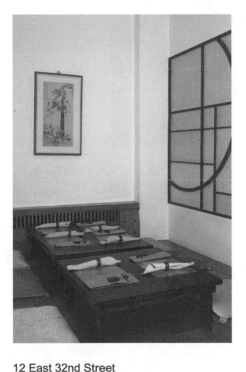

12 East 32nd Street
New York, NY 10016
T.212.213.0077
F.212.689.0780
info@hangawirestaurant.com
www.hangawirestaurant.com

HANGAWI

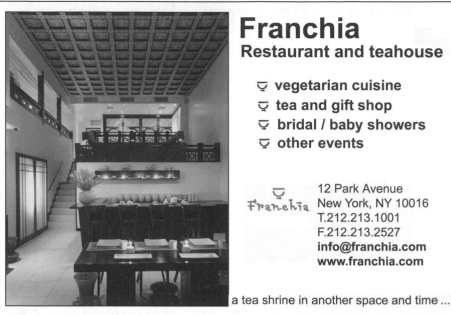

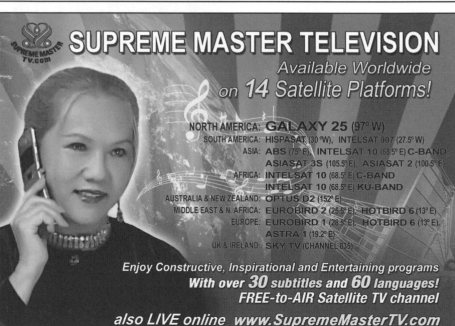

CONTENTS

Appreciations

"More than a food guide, a portable conscience. "

New York Times

"The Vegan Guide to New York City is a very complete Guide!"

The New York Daily News

"Packed with information and insightful commentary, THE VEGAN GUIDE TO NEW YORK CITY invites you to take a juicy, cholesterol-free, cruelty-free bite out of the Big Apple.

Michael Klaper, M.D.
Author, Vegan Nutrition: Pure and Simple

"Indispensable for the traveling vegan, this guide will most definitely enhance the vegan experience in New York. As a long-time resident of this city, I learned a great deal!"

Gary Francione, Professor of Law, Rutgers University
Director, Animal Rights Law Clinic

"Also, order a copy of the book, *The Vegan Guide to New York City*, and don't forget to pack it with you on your trip (along with this post)!"

PETA PRIME TRAVELER

A WORD FROM THE AUTHORS

We love food. Whatever image the uninformed may hold of vegans as joyless ascetics who subsist on carrots and brown rice, it certainly does not hold true for us. We love to eat from a world of varied cuisines—a simple macrobiotic meal of miso soup and steamed vegetables one day, a sumptuous Italian feast of grilled pizza with roasted sweet peppers and portobello mushrooms the next, a rich Thai or Indian curry dinner the third—and one of the joys of New York City is that you can find them all within the same block. That's because New York is a world city.

The Vegan Guide to New York City was launched back in 1994, when Rynn Berry, Max Friedman, and Dan Mills, under the tutelage of Alex Bourke, author of Vegetarian London, put together the first slender edition. That same year Dan went back to London to practice law, and Max went to graduate school to get a Ph.D. in American History. That left Rynn Berry in New York City to carry on with the Vegan Guide. In the years since, Rynn has put out a new edition of the guide annually. In 2001, he joined forces with Chris Abreu Suzuki, and Barry Litsky to put out the first quality paperback edition of the Vegan Guide. Rynn, Chris and Barry met at the Farm Sanctuary, a refuge for farm animals in Watkins Glen, New York.

Rynn Berry is the historical advisor to the North American Vegetarian Society. He is the author of several seminal books on vegetarianism; they include The New Vegetarians, Famous Vegetarians and Their Favorite Recipes, Hitler: Neither Vegetarian Nor Animal Lover, and Food for The Gods Vegetarianism and the World's Religions. In 2004, Rynn was commissioned to write a 6,000 word entry on the history of vegetarianism in the US for the Oxford Encyclopedia of Food and Drink in America. In 2010 Rynn co-authored the book, *Becoming Raw*. Rynn contributes frequently to both scholarly and spiritual publications.

Chris Abreu-Suzuki, Ph.D., is a professor of Mathematics, a long distance runner, who has won many races, a fervent animal rights activist and a connoisseur of vegan food. She's been a vegan since 1992 and an ethical vegetarian since 1977.

Barry Litsky, an intellectual property lawyer, who lives in New York City, does pro bono work for animal rights causes. He is also a vegetarian gourmet, who loves to whip up vegan meals for friends in his apartment.

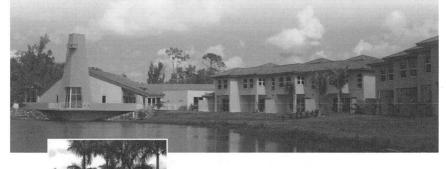

A FEW NOTES ON DINING IN NEW YORK...

There are more than 100 restaurants described in this book, but by no means should you limit yourself to them. New York is a city where you have the wide world at your doorstep, and you should not hesitate to plunge right in. All the restaurants listed in this guide offer vegan meals, but vegans will also do well at restaurants that do not go out of their way to cater to them, bearing in mind a few basic principles.

There are two centers for Indian food in town. One is 6th Street between 1st and 2nd Avenues, a block known as "Little India" for its cheek-by-jowl Indian restaurants. The joke is that there's one kitchen and a conveyor belt. Less well known to tourists is the community on Lexington around 28th Street, where the patrons are often Indian, too. As a rule, you should ask if they cook with ghee (clarified butter). We've listed Indian restaurants that use oil in most of their dishes, but ask anyway. You can request that they leave off the raita (yogurt with cucumbers).

There has been a boom in the popularity of Mexican food in the United States in the past few years, notably when salsa bypassed ketchup in condiment sales. In Mexico, Mexican food is based on corn or wheat with beans, but prepared with lard, cheese and meat stock, making strict vegan travel there a challenge. In New York City, there are a few authentic and many cheap Americanized places to eat Mexican food unsuitable for vegans. However, the last five years has seen an explosion in the number of trendy, "Cal-Mex" or "Tex-Mex" or "San Francisco Style" restaurants serving a healthy variation of Mexican cuisine prepared without lard, containing fresh vegetables and usually with the option of soy cheese, whole wheat tortillas and brown rice. (Almost all soy cheeses contain casein, a milk derivative; most tofu sour cream does not. See Glossary.) We have included addresses for these chains of healthy, vegan-friendly Mexican restaurants, where some of the best meals in the city are to be had. While they are similar, we give Burritoville a slight edge over the others:

Some of the most talented chefs in town are at moderate to expensive Italian restaurants. Vegans can always find something to eat here, if you request that your food be prepared with olive oil instead of butter, and make sure they leave out the common flavorings of Parmesan cheese and prosciutto (ham). Fresh pasta is often, but not always, made with egg. At Thai restaurants, it's dried shrimp and fish sauce you want to look out for. But we should offer this caveat: Since non-veg restaurants use utensils and working surfaces that may have come in contact with animal flesh, it is always preferable to eat in vegetarian/ vegan restaurants to avoid cross-contamination. Now go ahead and explore.

Nearly every restaurant in this guide offers take-out (meals to take home) and almost all of them also will deliver food right to your door, if you're in the area (say, within fifteen to twenty blocks). Because this service is nearly universal, we have specified only when a restaurant does NOT deliver or serve take-out. Otherwise, if the weather's bad or you'd rather stay indoors, you can call any one of these places and have your dinner in the comfort of your own room. Delivery is almost always free, usually with a minimum total order of $7-12, and you should tip your delivery person 15% of the bill. You can simply call up and tell them what you want, or ask what they have without meat or milk products; or, better still, do as New Yorkers do and start

Think. Create.
Explore. Celebrate.

For twenty-five years, CAF has supported thinkers
and researchers, artists and authors whose
work expresses a positive concern for all animals.

Through music, dance, film, poetry and philosophy
we explore issues, foster dialogue and build a deeper
appreciation of human-animal relationships.

View our recent grant recipients at:
www.cultureandanimals.org

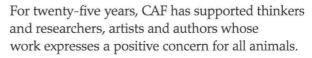

Culture & Animals
FOUNDATION

Tom Regan, President

Advancing animal advocacy through intellectual
and artistic expression.

your own collection of take-out menus from your favorite restaurants .

Most health food shops offer an assortment of ready-to-eat foods for vegans—hummus sandwiches, nutburgers and salads—in the refrigerator case. These tend to be OK, range in price from two to four dollars and can be just the thing if you want a quick snack. We've made a note by health food shops that go a little further, with a fresh salad bar, sandwich counter or buffet.

More and more liquor stores in New York stock organic wines, and of these, several labels are vegan—they use no fish or eggs in the "fining" (clarifying) process. Look for anything by the Organic Wine Works label or anything by Frey except the 1991 Cabernet, which was fined with egg whites. If you can't find them anywhere, try Warehouse Wines and Spirits at 735 Broadway (at Astor Place) or the slightly more expensive Astor Wines and Spirits at Lafayette and Astor.

An important note for our foreign readers: tax and tip are NOT included in the price at American restaurants, so figure on adding another 8.65% for the city and 15
20% for the service. American servers get paid an abysmal hourly wage and earn most of their salary from tips, so this is not really optional: unless you get terrible service, everyone leaves 15% as a matter of routine, and it's nicer to leave 20%. An exception is when there is no server, as in buffets or self
serve cafeterias; and when you dine in a group of more than five persons, the tip ("gratuity") may be figured into your total. People who deliver take-out to your door should also get a 15% tip.

A valid current Student I.D. will get you 10-15% off at many restaurants and some shops. The restaurants are grouped by neighborhood, and listed alphabetically within each neighborhood.

A NOTE ON OUR POLICY OF RESTAURANT SELECTION:

In 1994, when we first launched this guide, the number of vegan and vegetarian restaurants were rather sparse; so we included some vegetarian friendly restaurants that served some meat, but went out of their way to accommodate vegetarians. As of 1996, it was our feeling that we should no longer include any restaurants that served animal flesh of any kind--be it fish or fowl, snail or cow--because all restaurants have become friendlier to vegetarians; so to continue to feature vegetarian friendly restaurants in the Guide would make it meaningless. The vegetarian friendly restaurants that were included in the original guide were grandfathered in and phased out as they closed. In a few instances, restaurants started out as being vegan, then started serving increasing amounts of meat. These were so egregiously non-veg. that we had to delete them from the guide. But from then on, only vegetarian and vegan restaurants were to be included. That's why you may not find the trendy almost-vegetarian restaurant that you've been hearing about. Look to the conventional guides for those. Furthermore, in rating and ranking restaurants, we add and subtract points depending on how vegan they are. In other words, if they use honey or dairy products in their dishes, they will be penalized for it.

THE RESTAURANTS

ve=vegan
v=fleshless with vegan options
AE=American Express
MC=Mastercard
V=Visa
D=Discover

Full service means waiters take your order and bring your food. Counter service means you order at the counter and carry your meal to your table (these are usually cheaper, more casual places, often with paper plates). Prices listed are for typical vegan entrees. Address is listed opposite restaurant name. Nearest cross-streets are under address for easy location.

$ indicates an inexpesive entree

$$ indicates a moderately priced entree

$$$ indicates an expensive entree

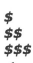 Indicates we especially recommend this restaurant for the quality of the food.

HARLEM
(North of Central Park)

CAFE VEG [ve] **$**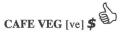

Full service   2291 Seventh Avenue
West Indian   bet. 134th/135th Streets
No cards   212-491-3223
No alcohol   M-Th 11am-9pm
                                F, Sa 11am-10pm

The rasta chefs at Veggie Castle in Brooklyn, and the Uptown Juice Bar in Harlem, were the first in the city to serve tasty vegan fast food with a Caribbean fillip. So it's great to see that Veggie Castle has just opened a branch in Queens, and that the Uptown Juice Bar has just opened this sister restaurant on 135th Street. We swilled the Mock BBQ Chicken Wrap served with Goddess Dressing, plus three sides--Okra, Collard Greens and Mashed Potatoes in just a few minutes. Then we slurped their tonic juices. The sharp-eyed waitress looked at us a touch disapprovingly, we thought, as we tottered out the door. True: we had eaten with unseemly gusto. But that's how we behave when we're around delicious Ital food.But wait, isn't that a pleonasm?

STRICTLY ROOTS [ve] $$ 👍

Counter service	2058 Adam Clayton Powell Blvd.
West Indian	at 123rd Street
No cards	212-864-8699
No alcohol	M-Sa 12pm-11pm
	Su 12pm-10pm

As the Rasta chef says, there is nothing served here that "crawls, walks, swims or flies." The menu changes every day and consists of items like broccoli & tofu, chick pea stew, seitan, falafel, tofu tempura, or veggie duck. The daily staples include millet, brown rice, greens and fried plantains. You can order small, medium or large portions of any combination of the above for $5, $7.50 and $10 respectively. Don't expect gourmet presentation, but it's good, wholesome stuff. They also have a variety of smaller dishes (e.g. veggie burger, vegetable salad) and beverages—juices, soy milk, and non-alcoholic ginger beer.

UPTOWN JUICE BAR[ve] $

Counter service	54 West 125th Street
West Indian	bet. 5th & Lenox
No cards	212-289-9501
No alcohol	daily 8am-10pm
www.uptownjuicebar.com	

A cross between a small cafe and a juice bar, Uptown Juice Bar is to be prized as much for its food as for its juices. Along with an array of juice combinations and smoothies, it serves delicious Caribbean-style vegan food. And although the menu contains alarming words like beef and fish, these are to be understood as "mock beef" and "mock fish." For instance there is a "turkey" salad, a "chicken" salad and a "fish" salad, but no turkey, chicken or fish died to produce these dishes. They're entirely ersatz and are very tasty. We had one of their combination meals that consisted of collard greens, tofu with black mushrooms, and a vegan shepherd's pie. To wash down this delectable grub, have one of their fruit smoothies or a juice tonic that is designed to cure whatever ails you. For impotence, drink a potent brew of carrot, parsley, cucumber, orange, and papaya juices. For asthma, gulp down a beverage containing carrot, celery, and grapefruit juice. Of course, if you're a vegan of long-standing, you probably don't have any of these ailments, so toast your good health--and your good fortune in being a vegan-- with a fruit smoothie instead.

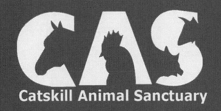

Catskill Animal Sanctuary

Meet Our Critters!
Sanctuary tours on weekends April - October

Cook With Our Vegan Chef
cooking classes year-round

Hold Your Special Event
vegan celebrations on the farm

Spend the Night
lodging in our 18th century farmhouse

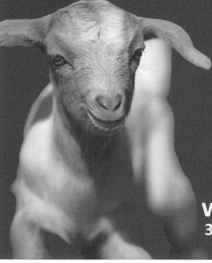

"Animals don't just live safely at CAS; they live joyously."
Wayne Pacelle, President, HSUS

www.CASanctuary.org
316 Old Stage Road
Saugerties, NY

UPPER WEST SIDE
(West 59th Street and Above)

AYURVEDA CAFE [v] **$$**

Full service
South Indian
All cards
No alcohol

706 Amsterdam Avenue
at 94th Street
212-932-2400
daily 11:30am-10:30pm

With its mango-hued walls and mottled sky blue ceilings, the Ayurveda Cafe resembles nothing so much as a film set for an early Merchant-Ivory movie, like Shakespeare Wallah or Bombay Talkie. So, it's not surprising to learn that the owner, Tirlok Malik, is a film director, who has parlayed a side interest in Indian cuisine into what seems to my taste buds to be one of the best Indian restaurants in town. Part Ismail Merchant, part Deepak Chopra with the Chopra ascendant, Malik has based his restaurant's dishes on the teachings of one of the four sacred books of Vedic Hinduism, which dates back at least 3,000 years--the Ayurveda (which means "knowledge of life" in Sanskrit.) Essentially, Ayurvedic cuisine tries to combine the six tastes, sweet. sour, salty, astringent, bitter and pungent, in order to produce a cuisine that is properly balanced for your body type. It certainly was right for my olfactory type. The Thali that I tasted was lightly spiced and lightly cooked so that you could taste each vegetable. I had to skip the raitas and desserts because they all contained dairy products and /or honey. Otherwise, a vegan can dine very handsomely here.

BLOSSOM DU JOUR UPPER WEST [ve] **$$** 👍

Counter servicr
Organic vegan fast ;food.
V, MC
No alcohol
www. Blossomdujour.com

165 Amsterdam
bet. 67/68 Streets
212-799-9010
daily 8:30am-10pm

See Description under Midtown West

 Indicates we especially recommend this restaurant for the quality of the food.

BLOSSOM UPTOWN CAFÉ [ve] $$$ 👍

Full Service
Global vegan, orgainc
All cards
Orgainc beer & wine
www.blossomnyc.com

466 Columbus Avenue
bet. 82nd/ 83rd Streets
212-875-2600
daily 11:30am-10:30pm

See description under Midtown West

CAFE VIVA [A.K.A. VIVA HERBAL PIZZERIA [v] $ 👍

Counter service
Italian vegetarian, kosher
All cards
No alcohol

2578 Broadway
bet.97th//98th Streets
212-663-8482
daily 11am-11pm

The founder, Tony Iracani, tells us that Cafe Viva is the only Italian vegetarian restaurant in the US, which after sampling the vegetarian antipasto and the tasty cheeseless pizzas, strikes us as shameful. Italian restaurateurs should beat a path to Cafe Viva to see how vegan Italian food is done, then go forth and do likewise. We had the Pizza Pura, a dairy-free, yeast-free spelt crust, topped with tofu marinated in Miso, grilled veggies and spinach with a vegetarian antipasto on the side. The fridge is stocked with healthful sodas such as Twisted Bean Vanilla Brew, Borealis Birch Beer, Ginseng tonics and China Cola. Recently Cafe Viva has expanded its menu to include a super anti-oxidant pizza; a Zen pizza, which features a green-tea herbal crust; tofu marinated with herbs, and a green tea pesto; it is topped off with a layer of maitake and shitake mushrooms. Another favorite is the Santa Rosa, which consists of a whole wheat crust layered with tofu marinated in miso, and topped off with sun-dried tomatoes and roasted garlic. Viva offers two types of vegan Lasagna as well as vegan Calzones made from spelt and whole wheat. Other pastas such as Raviolis, Strombolis, and Zitis are made from scratch and can be veganized to order. The service staff is friendly and helpful without being obsequious. One of the great pleasures apart from the food is that one can sit and read a paper or chat with a companion for hours without being hurried or pressured. We say, "Viva! Cafe Viva!"

HUMMUS PLACE/ V [v] $

Full Service
Israeli vegetarian, kosher
HUMMUS PLACE III [v] $

2608 Broadway
bet. 98th/99th Streets
212-222-5462

Full Service
Kosher Israeli hummus house
All cards
Wine & Beer

305 Amstardam Avenue
bet. W. 74th/ W. 75th Streets
212-799-3335
M-Su 10am-12am

See description under Greenwich Village, and other location under East Village, and Upper West Side.

MAOZ II [v] $

Counter service
Israeli falafel shack, kosher
All Cards
No alcohol
www.maozusa.com

2047 A Broadway
bet. 70th/ 71st Streets
212-362-2622
daily 11am-12am

See description under Midtown East and other locations under Midtown West, and East Village.

PEACEFOOD CAFÉ [ve] $$

Full service
Vegan world cuisine
All cards
No alcohol
www.peaceefoodcafe.com

460 Amsterdam Avenue
@ 82nd Street
212-362-2266
M-F 10am-10pm
Sa, Su 8am-11pm

We first met Eric when he was training to be a chef at the late-lamented vegetarian restaurant, Urban Spring, in Fort Green, Brooklyn. It was in the winter of '09 and Eric told us that he planned to sell his wildly successful antiques business in Soho and open a vegan restaurant to promote world peace. Eating vegan food, Eric opined with missionary zeal, is conducive to world peace. [Hence the name of his café—PeaceFood.] To be candid, it struck us, at the time, as being a mite quixotic, not to say hopelessly naive. But here we are, only nine months later--a proper interval for gestation--seated at tables in Eric's spiffy new Peacefood Café. It is tastefully decorated with a scattering of antiques--like the Victorian bakery display case that now doubles as a bookcase for vegan books—from Eric's old store. Not only is the food impeccably ethical and vegan, but it is also superbly prepared.

A disciple of the Supreme Master Ching Hai (an amalgam of Christianity and Buddhism founded by former Vietnamese nun, Suma Ching Hai), Eric and his partner, Peter, adhere to the first precept of Buddhism:, which is *ahimsa* [non-violence to all living creatures]. Eric has even gone to the length of inventing a cashew-based vegan substitute for the Roasted Japanese Pumpkin Sandwich. (The roasted pumpkin is mashed with a little sea salt, ground black pepper, and extra virgin olive oil, topped with caramelized onions, ground walnuts, vegan goat cheese, and seasonal greens.) He imported this sandwich--which was originally made with goat cheese-- from the menu of his former employer, the aforementioned, now defunct, Urban Spring.

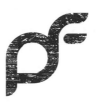
We started with the The Other Caesar (crisp romaine lettuce, tomatoes, smoked tempeh, red onions and crostini). It was so yummy that we instantly nominated it as best vegan salad of the year! [See Best Vegan Bites.] The Asian Greens (seasonal baby Asian vegetables, nixed sprouts, shredded carrots, tomatoes, marinated and baked tempeh, ground peanuts in a garlic, ginger, ponsu, and sesame dressing)--was a close runner up.

With my partner, Chris, I split a Pan-Seared French Horn Mushrooms Panini. Chris had to restrain me from nominating it as best sandwich of the year, as she felt we were showering Peacefood with too many accolades. Last year's best sandwich of the year is on the menu, as Eric also imported it from Urban Spring.

Next we supped on pizzas—Roasted Potatoes Pizza (with sautéed mushrooms, oil-cred blck olives, and truffle oil); and Mushroom Quxelle Pizza (with roasted sweet peppers, onions. and zucchini). This time we could not but concur--the mushroom pizza was absolutely tip-top. So in our Best Vegan Bites section, you'll find it listed as best pizza of the year.

For dessert we reveled in the raw Key-Lime Pie, which we followed with soy cappucino sweetened with agave nectar. It was the prefect coda to a peace-promoting meal, putting us in mind of a variant on a lyric from a John Lennon song—"All we are saying is give Peacefood a chance."

SOOMSOOM) [v] $

Counter service
Israeli falafel shack
All cards
No alcohol
www.mysoomsoom.com

533 West 72ng Street
bet Amsterdam' Columbus
212-712-2525
Su-Th 10am-11pm: F 10am-7pm

It looks as though the vegetarian falafel shack may soon displace the hamburger hut as New York City's fast food joint of choice. [To that eventuality, we say, in the immortal words of Ali Baba, "Open sesame!"] Soomsoom, which means "sesame" in Hebrew, is the newest manifestation of this trend.

The falafel balls here are bursting with flavor; they have a crisp brown jacket that conceals a moist, green chickpea and cilantro mixture. By the bright, bubbly ladies who work behind the counter—(one of whom was a vegan)--falafels were stuffed into a pita pocket that was artfully sauced with tahini. We then took our pita pockets to the salad bar and crammed them with chopped cucumbers, chopped tomatoes, a vegan cabbage slaw, and sealed them with a diabolic hot sauce. My friend had a side order of Sweet Potato Fries, which set off the Falafel sandwich quite nicely.

Vegans will of course eschew the Shakshuka Plate (a tomato stew of which the egg is an ineradicable ingredient;) the Sabich (a huumus and eggplant sandwich that may be ordered without the egg).

Perched precariously on stools in front of Soomsoom's storefront window—[All the other seats were taken.]--we sipped a mint lemonade. Then we gazed at the passersby as we savored our falafel sandwiches, trying to protract the taste sensation as long as possible.

ZEN PALATE- UPPER WEST SIDE [v] $$

Full service
Asian vegetarian
All major cards
No alcohol
www.zenpalate.com

239 West 105th Street
at Broadway
212-222-2111
daily 11:30am-10:45pm

See description under Midtown West and other locations under Midtown East and Midtown West.

 Indicates we especially recommend this restaurant for the quality of the food.

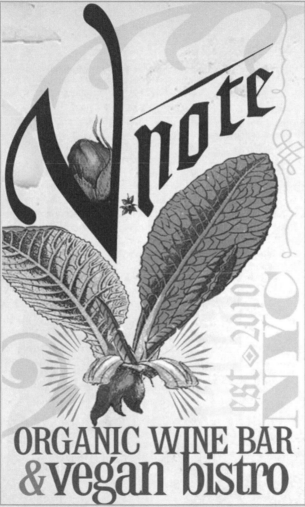

ORGANIC WINE BAR
&vegan bistro

1522 First Ave, NYC (between 79th & 80th Sts.)
212.249.5009

UPPER EAST SIDE
(East 59th Street and Above)

CANDLE CAFE [ve]$$$

Full service
Vegan, organic
All cards
Organic wine and beer
www. candlecafe.com

1307 Third Avenue
bet. 74th/75th Streets
212-472-0970 & 472-7169(fax)
M-Sa 11:30am-10:30pm
Su 11:30am-9:30pm

Back in the days when Bart Potenza, Candle's tousle-haired founder, ran a juice bar called the Healthy Candle, he dreamed of owning a vegan restaurant. A few years later, he realized his dream when he opened Candle Cafe. *Eighteen* years later, Candle Cafe has metamorphosed into one of New York's most popular eateries where celebrity watchers can spot environmental- and health-conscious actors like Woody Harrelson, and Alicia Silverstone, or prominent Animal Rights activists like Eddy Lama of The Witness , or Harold Brown of The Peaceable Kingdom.They come here because Bart and his partner, Joy Pierson, have a history of supporting environmental and animal rights causes and because they serve up some of the tastiest vegan food in town. We found just about everything on the menu appetizing, but our particular favorites were as follows: Our favorite appetizer was the Seitan Chimichurri (South American marinated seitan skewers with creamy *citrus-herb* sauce.) Our favorite entree was the *Sesame Crusted Tofu, served with black rice pilaf, steamed greens and saut ê ed gingered vegetables and a green coconut curry sauce.* We also relished the Tuscan Lasagna with sautéed green, Tofu-Basil Ricotta, and Seitan Ragout with a Truffled Tomato Sauce. For dessert, we fell upon the Chocolate Mousse Pie and the Decadent Chocolate Cake with Chocoalte Frosting. When it comes to Seitan dishes, which are the forte of both Candle Cafe and Candle 79, no other restaurant can hold a candle to the Candle. Also look for Candle Cafe Frozen Entrees at Whole Foods Market nationwide, and the Candle Cafe Cookbook, wherever books are sold.

CANDLE 79 [ve] $$$

Full service
Global organic vegan
All cards
Organic wines, beers and sakes.

154 East 79th Street
at Lexington Avenue
212-537-7179
M-Sa Lunch, 12pn-3:30pm
Dinner, 5:30pm-10:30pm
Su Brunch, 12pm-4pm
Dinner, 5pm-10pm

A special gluten-free menu is available. Private party rooms are also available.

New York's Upper East Side has a posh vegan restaurant serving Global Organic style vegan cuisine that can rival --in elegance and excellence- the best restaurants of the world.

.Bart Potenza and his partner Joy Pierson have transformed an unprepossessing two-story town house that was formerly a prosaic restaurant called the Dining Room into a restaurant whose interior design is as ravishing as are the dishes on its bill of fare. Start with a glass of organic Sangria at the intimate downstairs wine, sake, and spirits bar. With an extensive all-organic cocktail list, Candle 79's sleek and sexy bar is a popular spot for eco-chic dates!

At the table, begin with the Teaser: *delicious Saffron Lobster Mushroom Ravioli, with cashew ricotta, roasted tomato-truffle sauce, spinach, shallots and crispy capers.* Then proceed to the Wild Mushroom Salad with *Arugula,* Grape Tomatoes, Roasted Cippolini Onions, and Creamy Horseradish Dressing. Then on to the *main course* of *Caribbean Jerk Grilled Seitan, with brown ale-black bean sauce, plantains, collard greens, and mango-papaya salsa.* If you are a rawfoodist, try the wonderfully flavorful *Live Heirloom Tomato-Zucchini Lasagna.* Finish with the ever-addictive Chocolate-Peanut Butter Bliss- a creamy mousse confection nestled in a dark chocolate shell. Be sure to check the current menu on-line *(www.candle79.com)* as it changes with the season according to local organic produce. Much of the credit for Candle 79's dazzling menu is *owed* to head chef Angel Ramos, and pastry chef Jorge Pineda. We are avid fans of their seitan dishes both at Candle Cafe and at Candle 79. They have raised the preparation of Seitan to high art. Indeed, their Seitan Piccata (Sir Paul McCartney's favorite!)with Creamed Spinach, Savory Potato Cake and Lemon-Caper Sauce should make Seitan worshippers of even the most fundamentalist carnivore. Congratulations to Candle 79 for being named "Best Vegetarian Restaurant " in Zagat's 2007 and 2008, *and for their recent rave New York Times Review, in which Frank Bruni wrote that Candle 79 "showed him the light!"*Be sure to look for their latest stunning creation, the *Candle 79 Cookbook,* available wherever books are sold

GOBO [ve] **$$**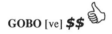

Full service
Organic, Asian-Western fusion cuisine
All cards
Organic beer & wine
www.goborestaurant.com

1426 Third Avenue
at 81st Street
212-288-4686
Su-We 11:30am-11:30pm
Th-Sa 11:30am-12am

See the description under East Village.

GREEN BEAN CAFE, THE [v] **$**

Counter service
Homestyle organic vegetarian
Visa & Mastercard
No alcohol
www. BeanGoneGreen.com

1413 York Avenue
bet. 75th/ 76th Streets
212-861-1539
M-F 7am-9pm
Sa, Su 9am-9pm

When we walked into the Green Bean, shortly after it opened, we saw three generations of the owner's family all of whom were vegetarian, all working behind the counter. There's Darrel the owner, Darrel's mother, Barbara, and Darrel's nephew, Nirmal. Darrel also owns the restaurant down the block called Beanochio. In fact, the Green Bean now occupies the space formerly inhabited by Beanocchio, which outgrew its space. That's what beans do; they grow and grow as if by magic.

As we know from *Jack and the Beanstalk,* beans have magical properties. And this Green Bean is no exception. Magical is it that such a small space can produce such a high volume of high quality dishes and beverages. Appropriately enough we started with a beany dish--their Spicy Tempeh with Mixed Greens and Sweet Potatoes. Superb! Next we tried their Seitan Cutlets with Mashed Potatoes and Miso Gravy. Pluperfect!

Their smoothies are made with organic frozen fruit and contain no added ice. (Most juice bars spike their fruit with superadded ice as a stretcher.) We quaffed the Berry Smoothie, and ii really socked our knocks off!

For dessert we munched cookies and cupcakes, which are all vegan, all delicious, and all baked downstairs in the basement. Needless to say, we left feeling satisfied and full of beans, magic beans

JUICE PRESS-3 THE [v] $$ 👍

Counter service	70 East 1st Street
Organic Juices and raw food	bet. 1st / 2nd Avenues/
All Cards	212-777-0034
No alcohol	daily 8am-8pm
Thejuicepressonline.com	

See description under East Village

PONGAL [v] $$

	1154 First Avnue
Full service	at 63rd Street
Indian vegetarian	212-355-4600
All majjor cards	Th 11:30am-10pm
No alcohol	F-Su 11:30am-10:30pm

See description under Midtown East.

SIMPLY PEELED) [v] $

Counter service	1371 Third Avenue
Soft serve shack	bet. 78th/ 79th Streets
All cards	212-794-2200
No alcohol	daily 11:30am-10:30pm
www.simplypeeled.com	

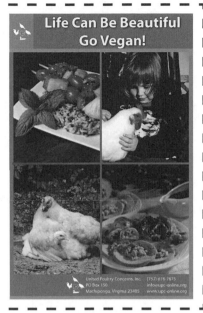

The four partners who own Simply Peeled were casting about for a healthy alternative to the malevolent iced glop served at the sleazy frozen yogurt shops and seedy ice-cream parlors that litter the Upper East Side landscape. Using a technique of their own devising, which combines pureed fruit, filtered water, and a hint of organic cane sugar---in their own kitchen, they concocted a sort of frozen sorbet that has the consistency of soft-serve ice-cream. They called it Fruizo.

Fruizo comes in three flavors—mango, banana, and strawberry. We had the Bandango Sundae (banana and mango fruizo, topped with tortilla chips, salsa and chopped mango bits). We also tried the Fruit Salad Sundae (banana, strawberry and mango Fruizo topped with berries, raisins, granola and cheerios.)

To be quite candid, we found the straight Fruizo to be somewhat bland; but when we added the toppings, the Fruizo came to life. There is a choice of 24 different toppings-only a few of which are non-vegan. The non-vegan toppings are the chocolate chips, which are made with milk, and the granola, which is made with honey. Fruizo is also used to make smoothies. We tried the Very Berry in which Fruizo is blended with blueberries, strawberries and raspberries.)

This was an appealing treat, but we had to expostulate to the counter person that we didn't want skim milk, or honey, or protein powders added to it. Although we much prefer the vegan ice-cream parlors like Stogo and Lula's Sweet Apothecary that are located in the East

Village, there is definitely a place for Fruizo in a neighborhood that is awash in frozen mammary secretion

V-NOTE [ve] $$$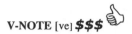

Full Service
Vegan Bistro & Wine Bar
All cards
Organic beer & wine
www.blossomnyc.com

1522 First Avenue
bet. 79th/ 80th Streets
212-219-5009
daily 11:30am-10:30pm

Just there short blocks away from Candle 79 , which it rivals in quality and service, is The V-Note a new deluxe vegan restaurant on the Upper East Side. It was started by Ronen Seri, the co-founder of Blossom. (In fact it is located on the site of the short-lived Blossom East.) So we were not too surprised to see some cherished items from Blossom show up on the menu.

V-Note is set in a rectangular shaped room with black walls adorned with large, colorful abstract paintings. All the tables were occupied when we arrived, so we were seated at the end of the bar where folks were sipping vintage wines and downing entrees rather than drowning their sorrows with booze. Case in point: We couldn't help noticing that the lady sitting to our left was sipping a Riesling while tucking into a Pasta Bolognese and perusing an article in the New Yorker on her i-pad.

Entirely vegan is the menu, and the wait staff! To a person, each waiter said, all unbidden, that he loved his job; liked working under Ronen; and wouldn't think of working anywhere else. We asked Chris, the headwaiter, to recommend an appetizer; he suggested the Cape Cod Cake. We were not disappointed. A piquant and flavorful cake composed of Yukon gold potatoes, black-eyed peas, and a chipotle aoli was set before us. We downed it with unseemly gusto.

Since we had done so well by Chris, we asked him to recommend an entrée. Medallions *Au Poivre,* he said unhesitatingly. [Seitan Medallions in a French peppercorn sauce are served with a cauliflauer-poatato puree, and steamed aasparagus.] They're so addictive that headwaiter Chris, who can select anything on the menu *gratis,* dines on them four times a week. We could easily see why. We tossed off the Medallions with a Calypso, a smoothie consisting of raspberry, pineapple, and banana. To be quire frank, most restaurant smoothies are execrable, but this one was worthy of Marcus Antebi's The Juice Press.

Also, on headwaiter Chris' recommendation, we wolfed the Wilted Spinach Salad with its soy bacon crumbles, roasted corn, shitake, tempeh and cashews, dressed with a balsamic vinaigrette.

For dessert, however, we decided to ignore Chris's recommendation of the Chocolate Ganache cake as being too redolent of Blossom, (where it is a cherished item on the dessert menu) in favor of the Fruit Tart, which was composed of three kinds of seasonal berries, topped *a la mode* with a scoop of soy vanilla ice-cream.

We were lucky to have dined at the V-Note on a Friday evening because there is live music on Fridays and Saturdays. An Argentine guitarist of no mean talent melts the house with his sultry licks. With the V-Note, owner Ronen Seri has struck just the right vegan note.

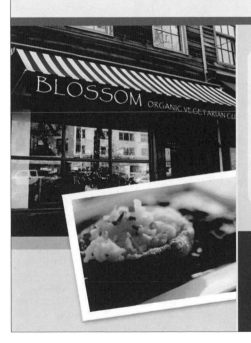

MIDTOWN WEST and Chelsea
(West 14th to West 59th Streets)

BLOSSOM DINING [ve] $$$ 👍

Full Service
Global vegan, orgainc
All cards
Organic beer & wine
www.blossomnyc.com

187 Ninth Avenue
bet. 21st/ 22nd Streets
212-627-1144
daily 11:30am-10:30pm

Erstwhile actors, Ronen Seri, and his wife Pamela, couldn't find a restaurant to satisfy their recherché vegan tastes; so they decided to open their own place. We vegan foodies are all in their debt. For now we have someplace to go besides Candle '79, on the upper east side, and Millennium, in San Francisco, to slake our appetite for organic vegan haute cuisine.

Indeed the restaurant's interior has a touch of the theater about it. With its chic townhouse setting; its cozy fireplace; its burnished wood tables; its floor-to-ceiling draperies; it looks like the perfect stage set for a posh restaurant

Despite their restaurant's high-toned elegance, Ronen and Pamela are not above stating, right on their menu, that "Blossom is first and foremost animal caring." Consequently, their "food is not only organic, it is also dairy and cholesterol free." This is the first time we know of that a restaurateur has had the courage to remind his/her patrons that conventional non-veg. food involves the wanton sacrifice of our fellow creatures.

We would eat at Blossom out of solidarity with Ronen and Pamela--just to pay tribute to their ethical approach to food preparation--but, fortunately, their food is so extraordinary that we also eat there for the sheer yumminess of the dishes.

Everyone we know. in our circle of vegan friends , raves about Blossom's appetizers--especially the South Asian Lumpia (curried seitan and potatoes wrapped in a crispy chickpea crepe, served with mango onion sambal). And, we are here to confirm that it, and the Black-Eyed Pea Cake (crispy cake of yukon gold potato & black-eyed peas, served with chipotle aioli) are as fresh and peppery as they're cracked up to be.

We're confessed seitan worshippers; so we reveled in the Barbecued Seitan Sandwich (barbecued seitan and caramelized onions with fresh cut fries or salad); and the Seitan Medallions (pan seared seitan cutlets served with herbed soft polenta and broccoli rabe). They would have delighted Old Split-foot himself, [who like most ungulates is doubtless a vegan].

For dessert we had the Chocolate Ganache Cake (a layered combination of rich chocolate ganache and chocolate cake). And the Pineapple Crepe (grilled pineapple wrapped in a crepe served with coconut reduction and green tea or vanilla ice-cream). It was a fitting climax to this play in three courses. We were chagrined--as with most extraordinary theater--only that it had to end.

Blossom Du Jour

Shrewd Fast Food – Prepared Vegan & Organic

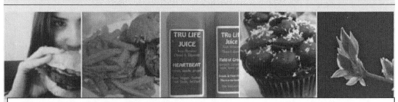

BLOSSOM DU JOUR [ve] $$ 👍

Full Service
Vegan fast ;food.
Cash only
Organic beer, wine & sake
www. Blossomdujour.com

174 Ninth Avenue
bet. 20th/ 21st Streets
212-229-2595
daily 11:30am-10:30pm

"Shrewd Fast Food" is how Pamela Elizabeth describes her latest addition to her expanding vegan restaurant empire—Blossom Du Jour. It could equally be described as "Gourmet Fast Food." Fast it assuredly was: We had to wait only four minutes for a savory Gluten Free Quesadilla (spicy black beans, corn vegan cheesse, and salsa) to appear; and Granny's Un-Chicken Pot Pie (savory un-chicken, carrots, corn, herbs, and spices) to emerge. Very tasty it was too. Our granny. were she still alive, would have adored it.

Our next order arrived a minute later. This was the Midtown Melt (cajun-spiced seitan, vegan cheese, agave guacamole, lettuce, chipotle aoli). My companion had the aptly named Skyscraper (vegan burger, soy bacon, vegan cheese, onion rings, lettuce, tomatoes, pickles, special sauce), which also scaled the dizzying heights of gourmet fast foodism.

All four dishes were worthy of the gourmet vegan fare at Pamela's three other eateries: Blossom. Blossom Café, and Cocoa V, not to mention her ex-husband Ronen's superb new vegan café, The V-Note, which has some dishes in common with the two Blossoms.

We consumed our meal while sipping chilled young coconut water, and gazing at the animal rights videos that were flickering on the video screen that is sunken into the wall above the small kitchen nook in the rear.

Blossom Du Jour occupies the former kitchen space of the adjacent Cocoa V. Since we are recovering vegan chocoholics, we were seduced by the aromas of vegan chocolate that wafted through the partition that separates Blossom Du Jour from a shrunken but still puissant Cocoa V. We fought the urge to conclude our very satisfying meal with some chocolate desserts at Cocoa V, but in the end gratefully succumbed.

COCOA V [ve] $$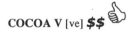

	174 Ninth Avenue
Full Service	bet. 20th/ 21st Streets
Vegan choolate, cheese, wine bar	212-242-3339
Cash only	M 1pm-8pm; Tu-Th 11am-9pm
Wine, beer & saake	Sa 10:30am-1qpm;; Su 12pm-8pm
www.cocoav.com	

"Blossom Village" is what Pamela Elizabeth's friends teasingly call the complex of vegan eateries that she owns between 20th and 22nd Streets on 9th Avenue. Diagonally across the street from the wildly successful Blossom is Pamela's new vegan dessert emporium called Cocoa V. The V is short for *vin*. The Cocoa stands for the exquisite vegan chocolates that her chocolatier has designed for the delectation of her clients. The chocolates are filled with vivid tasting centers such as caramel and raspberry ganache as well as crunchy roasted edamame, hazelnuts, and almonds. People normally order a selection of chocolates and accompany it with a savory dish like Pamela's tasty vegan quiche. Alternatively one may order a cheese plate which contains a wide array of vegan cheeses like a sun-dried tomato cashew cheese; or a kale-streaked cashew cheese. We're neither wine-bibbers nor beer drinkers so instead of imbibing, we chose to have an M-M-M-M Good, This is a delicious vegan hot chocolate laced with a jolt of espresso. Cocoa V is a dangerous place for recovering vegan choco-holics like us. The chocolates here, in their seemingly infinite variety, are so sumptuous and rich as to be addictive.

CRISP-2 [v] $

	110 West 40th Street
Counter service	bet. 6th Avenue / Broadway
Israeli-Indian falafel shack	212-661-0000
All major cards	daily 10am-10pm
No alcohol	Sa-Su 12pm-8pm
Eatatcrisp.com	

See description under Midtown West.

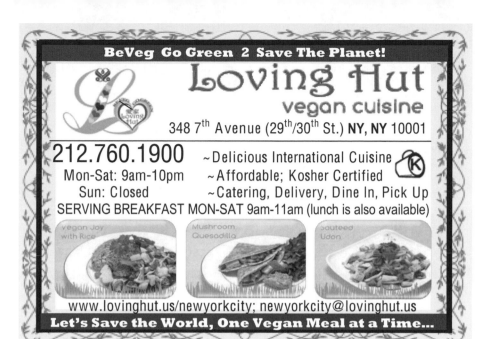
LOVING HUT [v] $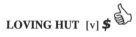

Full service	**348 Seventh Avenue**
Pan Asian	bet. 29th/ 30th Streets
All Cards	**212-760-1900**
No alcohol	M-Sa 9am-10pm
www.lovinghutnyc.com	Breakfast 9am-11am

With its 160 branches world-wide, [with one opening every month, and more than 60 in the pipeline], Loving Hut is the fastest growing vegan restaurant chain in the world. Recently, one opened in Paris, and we ourselves have visited the ones in Houston, and San Francisco. The globe-girdling vegan restaurant chain, which started in Taiwan in 2008, is the brainchild of t Chinese-Vietnamese lady who has founded a spiritual movement whose mission it is to promote compassion for animals and to save the planet.

At least two months before opening the restaurant., each franchise owner has to become a practicing vegan. Each franchisee is also responsible for developing its own menu. Consequently, the food at each Loving Hut is markedly different. Despite the diversity of menus, the food at each Loving Hut franchise is of a uniformly high quality.

We tried their Vegan Joy (Five grain rice mixed with vegan chicken and mixed vegetables.) and found it very much to our liking. Then we downed their generous Crispy Vegan Burger. (Tomatoes, pickled cucumbers guacamole, romaine lettuce, oatmeal vegetable patty, burger sauce on a whole wheat bun).It comes with a side salad and is their best-selling menu item.. We finished our meal with a tapioca pudding topped with fresh mango chunks. Simply felicitous! Ally, the manager, told us that Loving Hut is trying to lure people away from their meat-centered diet with delicious vegan food. Based on the gustatory delights that we sampled at Loving Hut, we would say they're succeeding admirably.

MAOZ IV [v] $

Counter service	200 W. 40th Street
Israeli falafel shack, kosher	at 7th Avenue
All Cards	212-777-0820

MAOZ V [v] $

Counter service	683 8th Avenue
Israeli falafel shack, kosher	bet. 43rd/ 44th Streets
All Cards	212-265-2315
No alcohol	daily 11am-12am
www.maozusa.com	

See description under Midtown East

MOSHE'S FALAFEL[ve] $ 👍

	Corner 46th Street
Food cart	at Sixth Avenue
Middle Eastern (Israeli), kosher	(no phone)
No cards	M-Th 11am-5pm
No alcohol	F 11am-3pm

Let's face it: most falafel places in the city are just plain "foul-awful!" Mainly, we think, this is because of the cross-contamination. All-too-often, the "foul-awfuls" in non-veg. places are deep-fried in the same rancid oil that is used to cook animal flesh. At this outdoor food cart, however--because the food is vegan and kosher--none of these concerns apply.

Perhaps it was psychological, but knowing that the falafels weren't contaminated made them taste that much better. Evidently, Moshe's customers concur, because when we sampled his food, there was a line around the block! Portions are generous. Topped with colossal pickles, stuffed with chunks of tomato, fistfuls of lettuce, and drenched with the obligatory tahini sauce, Moshe's Falafels are fully twice the size of the standard-issue falafel sandwich. For those who like their falafels hot, ask for a devilishly piquant hot sauce on the side. Or if you're traveling any distance before eating it, ask for the tahini sauce on the side too. [The trick to eating a falalel sandwich is to eat it on the spot lest the tahini sauce seep into the bread and make it soggy. And nothing tastes worse than a soggy falafel sandwich!] Moshe serves up an ample salad and a selection of vegan soups as well.

NATURAL GOURMET COOKERY SCHOOL [ve] *$$$*

	48 West 21st Street
Full service	bet 5th and 6th Avenues
Gourmet vegan	212-645-5170
All cards	F 6:30pm
BYOB	

Every Friday, the Natural Gourmet Cookery School has a feast that is prepared by the students at the school. The public is invited to partake of the students' cooking, which is vegan. Students, attired as waiters, serve four-course meals at large communal dining tables that are reminiscent of a college refectory. As in a college dining hall, the communal tables encourage the dinner guests to strike up conversations with total strangers, which adds to the convivial atmosphere.

The price for the four-course meal, at thirty-two dollars, is high, but then the cooking rivals that of any four-star restaurant. Truth to tell, we did overhear a few diners grumble about the meagerness of the portions. But the *nouvelle cuisine vegeterienne* style of cookery that is taught here dictates that portions be small. And the very fact that customers cry for more shows that the food is exceptionally tasty.

With the exception of only one item on the menu, we relished the food unreservedly. This was the Crispy Scallion Pancakes that were so crispy they tasted like hockey pucks. But the entree--Savory Baked Tofu Arame Stir-Fry with a Melange of Mushrooms and Fresh Vegetables in a Sweet and Spicy Sauce Served on a Bed of Lettuce and Crispy Rice Noodles--was divine. And the dessert! The dessert! Five Spiced Roasted Peach Pie with vegan Basil Ice-Cream and Sour Cherry Sauce, was sublime.

While everyone was clamoring for seconds and thirds on the vegan Basil Ice-Cream, the door to the kitchen suddenly swung open, and we saw something that we were not supposed to see. We spied the dessert chef downing a soup bowl filled with gobs of vegan Basil Ice-Cream. That's how good it was!

OTARIAN II [v] *$*

	947 Eighth Avenue
Counter service	at 56th Street
Global ovo-lacto vegetarian	212-875-2600
All cards	M-Sa 11am-11pm
No alcohol	Su 11am-10pm
www. Otarian.com	

First of all, it's Otarian, not Oatarian.. The "O" is meant to symbolize the *orbis terrarum*. It might also symbolize the first letter of the surname of Radhka Oswal, the Perth-based vegetarian entrepreneur who has launched a chain of vegetarian fast food restaurants with the object of lowering the planet's carbon footprint. To this end, all the furnishings are made from recycled materials. The eating utensils are compostable. There is an LED monitor that demonstrates how one's food choices impact the planet. By eating Otarian's Tex-Mex Burger, for instance, we are told that it is the equivalent of driving an eco-friendly car.

Unfortunately, their Tex-Mex Burger like so many other items on the menu is not vegan. This is where their "eco-friendly" menu verges on hypocrisy. Otarian could dramatically reduce its carbon footprint by removing eggs and dairy products from its menu and going vegan. Dairy cows are a major source of green house gas emissions. They liberate methane, which is one of the deadliest of the greenhouse gases. Moreover, dairy products are cruelly exploitative of cows and are agriculturally unsustainable—to say nothing of their being detrimental to human health. [See Dr. T. Colin Campbell's *China Study (passim)* and Dr. Caldwell B. Esselestyn's *Prevent and Reverse Heart Disease (passim).*] One of the few items on the menu that was vegan was the Spicy Vegetable Noodles, We ate them with gusto. None of the desserts was vegan; so we had to forgo it.

Mr. Barlow, the manager, told us that he was wary of vegans because not a few vegans, when they learned that the menu contained eggs and dairy products, turned on their heel and stalked out. Perhaps it may seem that we are being hard on this ovo-lacto vegetarian restaurant. But when they congratulate themselves on their low carbon footprint, while continuing to serve eggs and dairy, they invite unsparing scrutiny.

SUKHADIA INDIA PAVILLION [v] $$

Counter service	17 West 45th Street
Pan Indian	bet.5th/ 6th Avenues
All Cards	212-395-7300
No alcohol	M-Sa 9am-9pm
www.sukhadia.com	

As the brain drain from India has tilted towards New York, many Indian vegetarian restaurants have sprung up to cater to the tastes of Indian professionals--a preponderance of whom are lacto-vegetarians. "Lacto," unfortunately. is the operative word here. In the evening, most of the dishes are awash with milk, yogurt and cheese; which makes it difficult for the fastidious vegan. We asked the proprietor, Phil Sukhadia, if the chef could make vegan versions of the dishes containing cheese, ghee or yogurt. He said that he would gladly do so. But we had to wait half an hour for him to tell us that there were only two vegan dishes available--Chana Masala and Suki Bhaji. While these dishes were quite tasty, they were not the vegan versions of the Indian entrees that we had requested.

At lunchtime, there is a buffet, which appears to have more non-dairy dishes to choose from, but even some of these may be cooked with yogurt or ghee; so it pays to inquire of the chef or the sous-chef. Phil told us that there were so many Jain customers, who ply their trade in the nearby diamond center, that he had a special menu designed just for them. And, indeed, the Jain menu, which is a sidebar to the main menu, features a number of dishes that are specially prepared for their stringent dietary requirements. For instance, Jains do not eat root vegetables lest they kill the plant or disturb the microbial and insect life that dwell in the root system. Also, their religious dictates prohibit them from eating vegetable-fruits that contain a superabundance of seeds, such as eggplant, lest they ingest the seeds of life. However, poring over the Jain menu and seeing the number of dishes that contained cheese and milk, made us wonder if the vaunted Jain compassion for insects and microbes did not extend to the cow, which is milked remorselessly and whose unwanted male calf is callously turned into veal.

However, what struck us as most odd is that the restaurant should go to great lengths to please Jains, but not do anything to please vegans. Sukhadia's is one of the few Indian lacto-

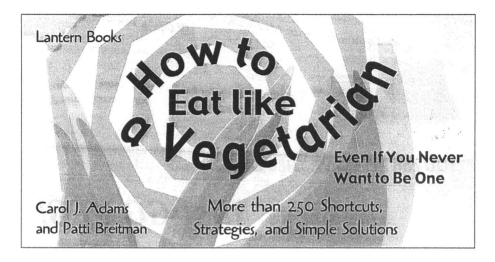
vegetarian restaurants in Manhattan that does not make some concessions to vegans. Madras Cafe for instance, marks vegan dishes with a "V" and has dishes that use soy foods, as does Desi Junction. New York Dosas, is the only Indian restaurant (actually a restaurant on wheels) that is 100% vegan. The desserts at Sukhadia's are almost all tainted with milk, cheese and ghee. Finally, the bill was twice what it should have been. So it definitely repays one's effort to examine one's bill, as well as the bill-of-fare, very, very carefully when dining here.

TERRI [ve] **$** 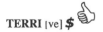   60 West 23d Street

Counter service   bet. Fifth/ Sixth Avenues
Vegan Café (kosher)   212-647-8810 ; 212-213-6068
All major cards   M-F 6am-11pm
No alcohol   Sa,, Su 8am-4pm
www.Terrinyc.com

Location is everything in the restaurant biz, and, in this respect, Terri is particularly well-favored. To the left, as you enter, it is flanked by an apartment building and to the right, it is flanked by a branch of HRC, In fact as we were downing our sandwiches, svelte ladies in leotards, who had just completed their gym workout strode in to slake their thirst with a juice cocktail; their hunger with a salad.

Founded by two former staff members off Blossom Uptown, Terri serves a delicious selection of vegan sandwiches, wraps, smoothies, as well as breads and baked goods that are baked on the premises. [Many of the baked goods are gluten free.] We shared a Roasted Vegetable Sandwich (eggplant, squash, sun-dried tomatoes, peppers, kalamata olives, and a dash of balsamic vinegar) served on Italian Rosemary Foccacio bread It was intensely flavorful. We followed this with a smoothie—The Brazilian Bombshell (Acai, acerola,,blueberry,.mango,,banana, soymilk.) It doubled as a delicious dessert.

Although Terri rhymes with berry, we were puzzled as to why a vegan restaurant should bear the name Terri. It turns out that the two owners, Mike and Craig, dubbed the restaurant, Terri because, by coincidence, both their mothers are named Terri With the high quality of the vegan food dished up here, Craig and Mike have done their respective Terris proud.

ZEN PALATE-HELL' S KITCHEN [v] $$ 🤏

	663 Ninth Avenue
Full service	at 46th Street
Asian vegetarian	212-582-1669
All major cards	daily 11:30am-10:45pm
No alcohol	
www.zenpalate.com	

This Zen Palate stands sentinel at the end of New York's restaurant row, providing the only palatable vegetarian option in the theater district. In the cozy, tastefully decorated interior, we love to dine on a pre-theater repast of Scallion Pancakes as an appetizer, followed by a main course of Mediterranean Medley (artichokes, basil, and tomatoes, stir-fried to perfection in a zesty garlic sauce). For dessert, it is our wont to have their scrumptious Chocolate-Raspberry Reincarnation. Now, properly fed, we're ready to watch the "strutters and fretters" on the boards of Broadway.

See other locationn under Midtown East and Upper West Side.

Indicates we especially recommend this restaurant for the quality of the food.

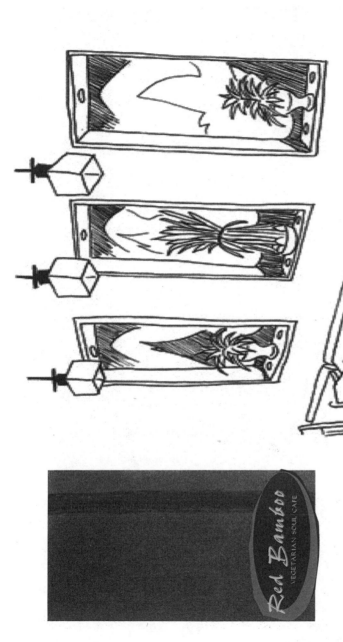

140 West 4th street

New York, NY 10012

1-212-260-1212

Red Bamboo
VEGETARIAN SOUL CAFE

MIDTOWN EAST and Gramercy Park
(East 14th to East 59th Streets)

BODY AND SOUL [v] **$**

Food stand
International, organic
No cards
No alcohol

Union Square Farmer's Market
at East 17th Street
212-982-5870
M, F 8am-6pm

One of the best ways to keep body and soul together in the city is to have a light vegan meal at the vegan food stand in the Union Square market, which is called aptly enough Body and Soul. Started by the owners of Counter restaurant back in 1994, it draws throngs of hungry folk for breakfast, lunch, early light suppers, and snacks. And it's not hard to see why. The out-size wraps and turnovers are quite toothsome. Try the Saffron Potato wrap which teases the palate with plantain chunks hidden inside. Or try the Spinach Portabello Turnover, which is filled with tofu ricotta, and tastes a bit like a Spinach Lasagna. You might want to complement this with a dairy-free Blueberry Muffin, or a Sweet Potato Muffin. Don't leave the stand without biting into a melt-in-your-mouth Chocolate Brownie, or a Wheat-Free Almond Cookie. Then repair to one of the benches in Union Square Park and have an al fresco meal.

See other location in Brooklyn.

BONOBOS [ve] **$** 👍

Self service
Organic living food, kosher
All cards
No alcohol

18 East 23rd Street
bet. Park Avenue/Broadway
212-505-1200
M-Sa 11:30am-8pm

A vegetarian oasis on the E 23rd Street fast food alley, Bonobos is a unique and delightful deli-style restaurant, serving mostly organic 100% vegan and 100% raw fruits, vegetables, nuts, and seeds. Dine on freshly made, tasty preparations under a huge skylight amid lots of plants. Or order lunch or dinner to go and take it to Madison Park across the street. In any event, the friendly staff will let you sample any prepared food to your heart's content. The prices are very reasonable and there is always a good selection of salads and fresh dressings, nut pates, soups, raw "ice- cream," puddings, and more. Everything is made on the premises with the freshest ingredients. Because Bonobo's food is not cooked it retains the maximum nutritional value and good taste.

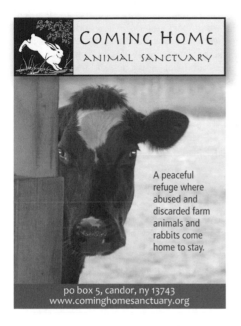
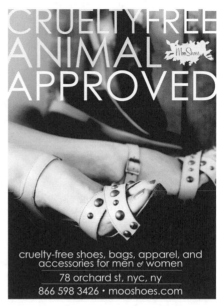
Bonobos are awesome healthy pleasure-loving primates who are closest to humans, closer than chimpanzees. Their natural, instinctive diet is primarily fruits vegetables nuts and seeds. Who needs the diet doctors? Bonobs's is kosher and is under strict rabbinical supervision

CHENNAI GARDEN [v] **$$**
Full service
Kosher South Indian / Punjabi
All cards
No alcohol

129 East 27th Street
bet. Park/ Lexington Avenues
212-689-1999
Tu-F 11:30am-10pm
Sa, Su 12pm-10pm

Back in the late 1980s, Pradeep Shinde and Neil Constance, the two owners of this Curry Hill eatery, were among the first to open a kosher Indian vegetarian restaurant in New York. They were so successful that they retired to Orlando to take a flyer in the resort hotel business. They were successful there too, but they found that they pined for the fast tempo of New York City. So much so that they decided to collaborate on another kosher Indian vegetarian restaurant-- despite the heated competition.

Their new joint venture is called Chennai Garden. The garden is a mere figure of speech (a row of plants that borders the front window), but Chennai is the pre-colonial name of Madras, the cultural capital of South India. And the restaurant breathes the pre-colonial spirit of South India before the Raj, when flesh food was an anomaly. Our palates were tickled by the Tamarind Pullao (rice perfumed with Tamarind and peanuts), the Bhindi Masala (okra curry) and the Behl Puri (a piquant mix of puffed rice, crisped noodles, onion and cilantro). In a nod to veganism, the Gulab Jamun, a flan which is usually made with powdered milk is made here with a powdered non-dairy mock milk. This makes Chennai garden the only Kosher Indian vegetarian restaurant where one may savor a vegan version of a traditional Indian dessert. The all-you-can-eat lunch buffet for $6.95 is one of New York's best restaurant bargains.

CRISP [v] **$**

Counter service
Middle Eastern
All major cards
No alcohol

684 Third Avenue
at 43rd Street
212-661-0000
daily 10-9

In this mid-Eastern vegetarian restaurant in mid-Eastern Manhattan, the word crisp is actually a euphemism for "falafel." Why substitute the word "crisp" for falafel? we asked the co-owner, Alan Kruvi, an Israeli, who was persuaded by his partner, Rakesh Barmecha, a Jain, to go veg. "Because falafels, as they are conventionally prepared, are greasy and low-end," says Alan. "Most falafel shops use the same oil. They never change it; they just add more oil to the original batch. We use fresh canola oil, and the oil is changed daily."

And lo it was true: the falafel sandwiches in this sleek falafel,..er "crisp" shack are wonderfully crisp and fresh-tasting. The Basic Crisp arrives packaged in a biodegradable box that is cinched with a pull tab. Pull the tab and the box disgorges an hygienic, delectable falafel sandwich.

There are multiple falafel or "crisp" sandwiches on offer. Unfortunately, the only one that vegans can eat is the Basic Crisp. That's because all the others –the Mexican, the Mediterranean, the Parisian--are suffused in sauces that contain insidious ingredients like butter, milk, and cheese.

On the other hand, the Hummus Bowls, of which there are five, are all impeccably vegan. We had the Hummus Bowl with Sautéed Mushrooms [a concave dish of snowy hummus with a huge dollop of sautéed mushrooms in the center] and was quite fetched by it. Others to choose from include Hummus Bowls with Sautéed Eggplant, with Israeli Salad, and with Roasted Pepper.

Blended teas, sweetened with agave nectar, are paired with each dish. As in all the other falafel shacks in the city, there is the obligatory fresh lemonade served with a sprig of fresh mint.

All the utensils are compostable and bio-degradable. So just by virtue of eating here, one may make an ecological as well as an ethical affirmation, which is gratifying to the conscience as well as to the palate.

FRANCHIA [ve] *$$$* 👍

Full Service
Korean –inspired Asian fusion
All major cards
Oriental & Western Wines, Beers &
Soju cocktails
www.Franchia..com/

12 Park Avenue
bet. 34th/ 35th Streets
212-213-1001
M-F 12pm-10pm
Sa,Su 1pm-10pm

Franchia is a vegan café, owned by William and Terri Choi, the people behind Hangawi, which Franchia rivals in elegance. Its name, Franchia, means "free, lavish, and generous." The interior space is nothing if not lavish. It is multi-tiered with a commanding ceiling. Decorated with colorful motifs, the ceiling is actually a replica of the ceiling from a Korean palace. Franchia is a refuge from the turmoil and hubbub of the city, where one may dine on delicious vegan fare in a Zen-like zone of tranquility.

Besides the wide selection of premium quality teas, Franchia also offers a delectable selection of vegan dishes comprising appetizers, salads, dumplings, noodles, wraps, bibimbap, stone bowl rice, main dishes and vegetarian sushis. Franchia's noodle dishes are especially interesting with selections such as sizzling spinach noodles, organic soba noodles, Spicy Franchia Noodles, and many more.

By the way, Franchia is *the* place to come for bibimbap (the internationally renowned Korean rice dish that is topped with a variety of zesty vegetables.) At Franchia one may order bibimbap in a variety of selections, such as avocado, tofu, and vegetarian "duck." These may be served in a stone bowl, or in a bibimbap version.

Franchia also serves a wide selection of exotic teas, many of which are purported to have medicinal powers. Try 1st Picked Korean Wild Green Tea from the rocky slopes of Mt. Jilee, or 2nd Picked Mt. Guhwa Green Tea. For those who prefer herbal teas, there is a Ginger Tea, a Date Paste Tea, Korean Plum Tea and an Organic Dandelion tea.

High tea is observed at Franchia. Between lunch and dinner, one may also enjoy a relaxing afternoon tea at Franchia: The Royal tea tray entitles one to a starter choice of tea and an appetizer tray presenting vegetarian dumplings, pancakes, vegetarian sushis, vermicelli spring roll, soy "meat" sticks, and mini tofu patties, a dessert tray of two mini desserts and a finale choice of tea.

With our Date Paste Tea, we ordered dinner that included an appetizer of their mouth-watering vegetarian dumplings. For a main course, we ordered the Tofu and Roasted Kabochah Pumpkin in sesame soy sauce with a side order of Avocado Bibimbap (Mixed rice wih avocado and vegetables served with bean paste sauce.) My partner had Soy 'Chicken' Sizzler on a Hot Plate with a side of Vegetarian 'Duck' in stone Bowl Rice, which she downed with gusto! For dessert, we had their incomparable Soy Cheese Cake with a dollop of Raspberry Sorbet. All of their dishes were exquisitely delicious and elegantly presented.

Franchia is also a popular place to hold bridal and baby showers. The bride-to-be is dressed in a traditional Korean bridal costume and shown how to brew tea in the traditional Korean way.

HANGAWI [ve] $$$ 👍

Full service
Korean
All major cards
Oriental and Western wines and beer
Soju cocktails
www.Hangawirestaurant.com

12 East 32nd Street
bet. Fifth/ Madison Avenues
212-213-0077 ; 212-213-6068
M-F Lunch: 12pm-3pm;, Dinner: 5pm-10:30pm,
Sat 1pm-10:30pm, Sun 1pm to 10pm

Unless you've spent time in a Korean Buddhist monastery run by Alice Waters, you've never had food like this before. Slip off your shoes and experience a truly transporting zen dining experience [Make sure you are wearing attractive, clean socks!] Enter a zone of absolute harmony with the sounds of rushing wind and water filling the air, and prepare to be enchanted by an exotic menu of Korean vegan dishes: Grilled Todok *(Codonopsi Lanceolata)* [mountain root strips grilled in ginger soy sauce]; Organic Zen Bibimbap [assortment of organic mountain vegetables and greens over organic brown rice with hot chili paste.];Pumpkin Porridge; Ginseng Salad with bean paste dressing; Royal Green Tea.

Perhaps the best way to experience the unique flavors at Hangawi is to order the Emperor's Tasting Menu which brings you a variety of exquisitely presented vegan dishes. The service is impeccable and a meal at Hangawi always leaves you refreshed and buoyant.

The dishes presented in the Emperor's Tasting Menu changes monthly showcasing new creations by the chef.

There is also a seasonal menu highlighting some of the produce that is available during a particular season for eg the Matsutake Mushroom in the fall. Hangawi has been voted top vegetarian restaurant as well as top Korean restaurant for many years in Zagat's surveys

The owners of this superlative restaurant, William and Terri Choi, are devout Buddhists who come by their ethical vegan philosophy naturally. They are noted for their support of vegetarian and animal rights causes as much as for their devotion to the highest standards in food preparation and service.

MADRAS MAHAL [v] $$

Full service
Indian vegetarian, kosher
Major cards
Beer & wine

104 Lexington Avenue
bet. 27th/28th Streets
212-684-4010
Su 12pm-10pm, F 11:30am-3pm
M-Th 11:30am3pm & 5:30pm-10pm

The menu asks for your patience since the food is freshly prepared. Maybe that includes scything the wheat for chapatis. At any rate, it took 45 minutes to get drinks and an hour for samosas which were hot and flaky, with the rich taste of freshly ground spices. After another half hour we got Kala Chana (black chick pea curry) and Sukhi Bhaji (potato stir fried with hot pepper, dry fruit and nuts). But we were cranky after waiting so long, and the dishes didn't measure up to our expectations, especially at nine dollars apiece.

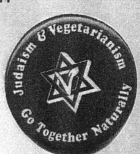
MAOZ I [v] **$**

Counter service	638 Union Square East
Israeli falafel shack, kosher	bet. 16th/ 17th Streets
All Cards	212-260-1988
No alcohol	daily 11am-12am

www.maozusa.com

Like a green shoot in a bowl of sprouting chick-peas, Maoz joins the other vegetarian falafel shacks in Manhattan--Crisp, Taim, Hummus Place, Moishes, et al, that have sprung up, seemingly overnight.

Oblong and solidly built, Maoz looks like nothing so much as a bunker, which is exactly what Maoz means in Hebrew. The "bunker" looks eminently capable of fending off carnivorous assaults from the malevolent fast food chains that huddle nearby. Maoz's secret weapon, with which, we predict, it will eventually flatten its carnivorous competitors, is the seductive flavor of its food. Another potent weapon is the undeniable fact that vegetarian fast food is healthful: It's the only fast food that isn't fat food. Rather, it's fit food. Eat as many salads and as many falafel sandwiches as you like and you'll still be slender.

All the food is prepared on the premises. The most popular item on the menu, which accounts for 80 percent of the sales is the Maoz salad, which one may assemble from as many as twenty healthful ingredients. Such as pickled eggplant, pickled carrot salad, couscous with parsley, shredded cabbage, onion and tomato salad, olives and, assorted pickles, special broccoli and cauliflower salads.

Add five falafel balls to the above ingredients, and you can construct a falafel salad. Add five falafel balls, and make yourself a Maoz falafel sandwich. We savored the Maoz Royal, which contained assorted salad ingredients plus eggplant and humus.

Bunkers and vegetarianism would seem to be incompatible notions, but, according to Nat Hirshman and his daughter. there are already 32 vegetarian bunkers in Europe. When you stop to consider it: a bunker is a zone of tranquility, an oasis of peace in a hostile world. And that's what Maoz is--a gustatory peace bunker that promises to spread and swallow New York.

See other locations under East Village and Upper West Side.

PONGAL[v] $$

	110 Lexington Avenue
Full service	bet. 27th and 28th St.
Indian vegetarian	212-696-9458
Major cards	M-Th 11:30am-10:30pm
No alcohol	F-Su 11:30am-11pm

Yes, the Big Apple boasts some of the finest Indian vegetarian cuisine this side of the Indus River. Night after night, one can eat in one great Indian restaurant after another without feeling that one has dined redundantly. The dining experience at Pongal is incomparable. Start with appetizers called Kachoori, then progress to a roll-your-own-crepe called Paper Dosa. This is a large Indian crepe made of rice flour and served with spiced potato on the side. The trick to rolling your own crepe is to tear off bits of dosa; fill them with the spicy potato mixture then dip them into a fresh coconut chutney. All dishes are served on banana leaves. Undhiya a Gujarati dish that we sampled is highly recommended containing as it does such exotic ingredients as yam, lotus root, potatoes and eggplant. When we'd polished off this and the okra-tomato curry, the waiter brought us Kachooris (deep-fried puffs of Toor dal lentil and Bathata Dada). We finished the meal with a decaf coffee from Madras. We forbore to have any of the tempting desserts as none (alas! alack!) was vegan. So we sauntered down to Stogo's for a vegan ice-cream.

See other location under Upper East Side.

PURE FOOD AND WINE (ve) $$$ 👍

	54 Irving Place
Full service	bet. 17th/ 18th Streets
Gourmet raw food	212-477-1010
All cards	M-Su 12pm-3pm
Organic beer & wines	M-Su 5:30pm-11pm

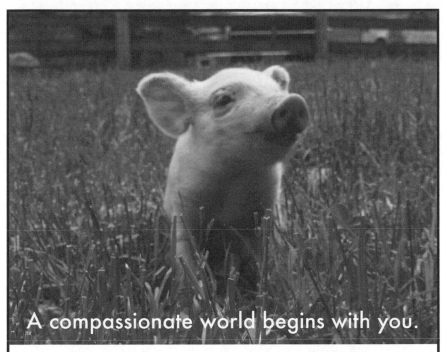
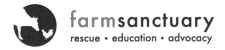

With the opening of Pure Food and Wine the preparation of rawfood has reached its apogee in New York, if not the world. The food, which is 100% vegan and raw, shows off the virtuosity of two talented New York chefs--Sarma Melngailis and Matthew Kenney (formerly of Matthews on the Upper East Side). In previous incarnations, both had won fame as chefs de cuisine cooking animal flesh for carnivores. But suddenly, about six years ago, over dinner at the rawfoods restaurant Quintessence, they had a simultaneous epiphany; they realized that eating vegan rawfood was better for their health, better for the health of animals, and better for the ecological health of the planet. Hence their motto, which they proudly display on the front page of their menu: "Handcrafted flavors that rejuvenate the body, mind, and planet."

A hard-bitten skeptic might scoff that chefs who excelled at making dead animal parts taste yummy should have no trouble infusing raw vegetable and fruit concoctions with flavor. Just so. This is why the food at Pure Food and Wine surpasses that of any other rawfood restaurant that we have visited. These two chefs have applied the *hautest* techniques of nouvelle cuisine to the preparation of rawfoods, and the results are truly sensational.

We can unreservedly recommend all the dishes that we tasted. Start with the Thai Lettuce Wraps that come with a spicy tamarind dipping sauce. Another appetizer to try is the Tomato Tartare with Kaffir Lime. For a main course, try the Beet Ravioli--[Rectangles of thinly sliced beets sandwiched together with a cashew nut filling]. Or the Golden Squash Pasta with Summer Black Truffles [Spiralized Yellow Squash slathered with a hearty truffle sauce with sweet peas and chervil]. For dessert, we commend to your tastebuds Chewy Dark Chocolate Cookie with Chocolate and Pistachio Ice Creams [This is a soft cookie, served with candied pistachios, strawberry sauce, and dollops of vegan ice-cream made from nut cream.]

The restaurant's interior is plush, and the walls are decorated with pictures of happy animals (pleased, no doubt, because they're not being eaten). The spacious patio is the perfect setting for the eating of things raw. Here one may dine al fresco, and in the event of a sudden downpour waiters are adept at setting up huge parasols that protect the diners from precipitation. The atmosphere is so convivial that strangers talk to each other across tables. Sitting next to us were two non-vegetarian women who were prolonging their meal by ordering endless glasses of coconut water and organic wine--because they couldn't tear themselves away from the place. It's that magnetic!

Not content to rest on their laurels, Kenney and Melngailis have collaborated on an uncook book, *Raw Food/ Real World: 100 Recipes to Get the Glow*, which tells one how to reconstruct the dishes that are on offer in the restaurant. Published by Regan Books, it became an instant bestseller. Early in 2006, Sharma and Matthew parted ways. Sharma continues to run Pure Food with her customary élan and Matthew has gone on to start a raw culinary school – cum-café in Oklahoma City called 100 Degrees Haute. He's also penned two more raw books: *Everyday Raw*, and *Entertaining in the Raw*.

PURE JUICE & TAKE AWAY [ve] *$$$*

Full Service
Gourmet raw food
$4.00-12.00 (all cards)
No alcohol

125 1/2 East 17th Street
bet. 3rd Avenue/ Irving Place
212-477-7151
daily 11am-11pm

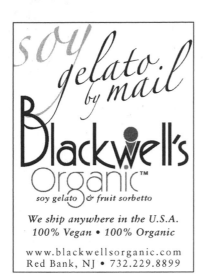
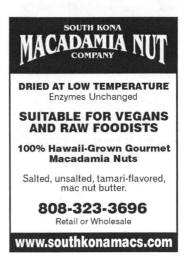
This is the vest-picket version of Pure Food and Wine with many of the menu items at PFW available for take-out. Here, you can get one of Pure Food's tastiest dishes, the Heirloom Tomato Lasagna with Basil Pesto and Pignoli Ricotta. Their Flatbread Pizza with Hummus, Avocado and Mint Pesto makes a delectable take away lunch, as does our favorite Tortilla Wrap with Chili Spiced 'Beans' The juice bar offers some exotic juice combinations such as Hot Pink (Beet Pineapple, Watermelon and Ginger) and smoothies. Try the Mango Shake (Mango, Fresh Coconut Water and a dash of Vanilla). Many of the desserts served at Pure Food are also offered here. We were glad to see the Toco Coco Brownies. And we also liked the Fruit, Granola and Vanilla Cream Parfait. The desserts, as at Pure Food, are made without honey. Making a commendable effort to be consistently vegan, they use Agave Nectar and Maple Syrup instead of honey.

SARAVANA BHAVANA (v) **$**

Full service
Chennai homestyle
$6.25-13.95 (major cards)
Wine & beer

81 Lexington Avenue
at 26th Streets
212-679-0204
Lunch Tu-Su 12m-4pm
Dinner 5:30pm-10pm

Saravana Bhavan--Englished means "house of Saravana". Brother of Ganesh, the elephant god of prosperity, Sarvana seems to be shedding a benign protection on this house. And according to the manager, Ms. Ramaya, they will need every ounce of Saravanaas' help. There is fierce competition with other Indian restaurants on Curry Hill, and there appears to be a jinx on the street corner where Saravanaas is located.. So far, every restaurant that has occupied this corner has failed.

But if the quality of the food and the service are anything to go by, Saravanaas will beat the odds. Already, the place is packed with frugal diners, both Indian and Western, who obviously recognize a bargain when they eat one. Modestly priced, and highly flavorsome, the cuisine--Chennai homestyle--is the type of food that one might encounter at a home in Chennai (formerly Madras). The menu abounds in delicious dosas, uthapams, vadas, and thalis redolent of India's deep south. Nearly all the dishes are cooked in oil, not ghee (clarified butter). But vegans must beware of the Iddly (Steamed Rice and Lentil Patty), which is topped off with a ladleful of ghee. Also, the Sambars in the Thalis are sometimes flavored with ghee.

For an appetizer, we had the Sambar Vada (Crispy Lentil Doughnuts in a Mild, Spicy South Indian Soup, Garnished with Onion and Cilantro). For the main course, we had the Dried Fruit Rava Dosa (a mildly spiced Crepe made of Wheat and Rice Flour, blended with Whole Raisins, Pistachios, and Cashews). This we dipped into three different coconut-based chutneys and a sambar. Verboten to vegans are the desserts. As in most Indian restaurants, they are highly caseous, containing ghee, milk, yogurt, and cheese.

Unlike other restaurants on Curry Hill, Saravanaas refuses to use frozen vegetables and will not serve leftovers. Ms. Ramaya told us that all the vegetables are purchased from local Indian suppliers. This accounts for the high quality and astonishing freshness of each dish. Saravana Bhavan is actually the New York branch franchise of a chain of successful Indian vegetarian restaurants that originate in Chennai. So all the dishes are made to standards set by the home office in Chennai. This can have its drawbacks. When we asked for soy milk to be used in a Lassi, or in an Indian coffee, which is pre-mixed with cow's milk, the manager told us that the home office does not permit its franchises to substitute soy milk for cow's milk. This strikes us as a silly practice-- especially as the home office has allowed the New York franchise to serve wine and beer, which no other restaurant in the chain is allowed to do. So, it is incumbent that vegans politely demand soy milk for their lassis and coffees.[If the Starbucks chain,--which is non-veg.-- can offer soymilk, then why not Saravana Bhavana, which is veg.?] Apart from this notable lapse, the service is faultless, and the food is very good value for the money.

TIFFIN WALLAH [v] **$**

Counter service

Mumbai homestyle

All Cards

Beer & wine

www.tiffinwallah.us

127 East 28th Street

bet. Park/ Lexington Avnues

212-685-7301

M-Su 11:30am-3:00am

M-Su 5pm-10pm

What is a tiffin wallah.? We asked Pradeep Shinde, owner of this eating establishment of the same name. An institution peculiar to Mumbai--which is where Pradeep grew up.--"tiffin wallah," is a man who fetches vegetarian lunches made by Mumbai housewives; he then ferries

them to their husbands in their city offices. Pradeep wanted to import this concept to New York in a slightly modified form. So he sees the restaurant as a sort of communal "tiffin wallah," conveying homestyle vegetarian meals to New York City's office workers.

Trained as an engineer in Mumbai, Pradeep moved to New York where he switched his major to hotel management at NYU. For a time, after his graduation, he worked as a personal butler at the Park Lane Hotel. Then, he started his own restaurant, Madras Mahal, which was the first vegetarian restaurant on Curry Hill. (Now there are seven.)

Tiffin Wallah hums with efficiency. Pradeep is everywhere at once, recalling his buttlilng days; he bustles about, overseeing the minutest detail. He wipes a spot of gravy from a bin cover, then he replenishes the salad bowls. A small but diligent wait staff is poised to do his bidding.

At lunch, the place is thronged with young, and middle-aged professionals who rhapsodize over the six-dollar buffet--the best luncheon deal in town. When we asked him how long he would peg the price at six dollars, Pradheep promised us, perhaps with a touch of hyperbole, that this price would be fixed in perpetuity.

On weekends, Tiffin Wallah serves exotic dosas (crepes) that cannot be found anywhere else. We recommend the Pesaratu, a dosa made from green lentils and green chilies; the Spring Dosa, which is a mixed vegetable dosa; and the Jaipur Masala Dosa.

At the buffet, we could eat only the Chana Masala, and a vegetable sabji. The other dishes, save for the delicious, small stuffed vegetable Uttapam, were caseous. Since many of our readers are persnickety vegans, as we are, they are reluctant even to eat in places where mammary secretions are served. So we extracted from Pradeep a promise that he would be willing to make mock meat substitutions for any caseous a la carte item. We urged him to visit Desi Junction, which, albeit a working-man's Indian restaurant, they nonetheless have integrated soy into a number of their formerly caseous dishes.

VATAN [v] $$$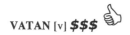

	409 Third Avenue
Full service	at 29th Street
Indian	212-689-5666 (reservations essential)
(V, MC)	Tu-Su 5:30pm-10pm
Full bar	Closed Mondays

At first glance, $31.00 *prix fixe* may seem like a lot of rupees, but think of a visit to Vatan as a cut-price ticket to India. The decor instantly transports you to a village in Gujarat, where costumed waiters and waitresses look as if they've just popped out of Aladdin's lamp to do your bidding. At the snap of your fingers, they will bring you all the appetizers you can eat; and the appetizers are so indescribably scrumptious, you'll eat yourself into a stupor. We stuffed ourselves unashamedly with delicate miniature samosas filled with peas and potatoes, the Chana Masala (chick peas with onions and coriander) and an array of Indian breads such as papadams and puris, but still found room for a rich dessert of Mango Rus (mango pulp). The music, authentic Indian ragas, is soft and unobtrusive. The food is prepared with canola oil, not ghee. The service is faultless.

The eating of animal flesh extinguishes the great seed of compassion

THE BUDDHA (SIDDHARTHA GAUTAMA OR SHAKYAMUNI)
563 BC–483 BC from *The Mahaparinirvana*

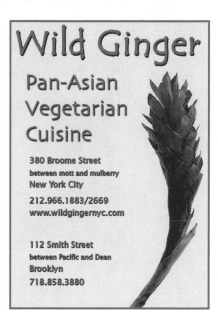

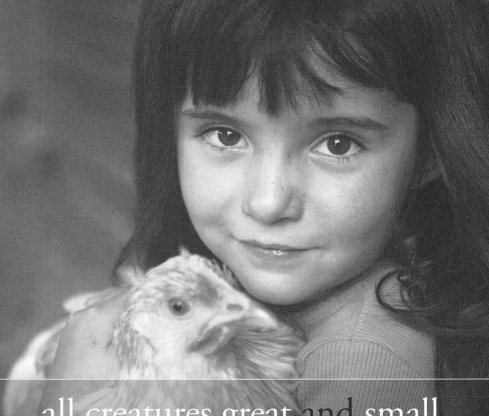

all creatures great and small

Millions of Americans love animals. But many creatures still suffer from cruel and abusive treatment.

Help us confront animal cruelty in all its forms. Visit **humanesociety.org** to find out what you can do.

Celebrating Animals | Confronting Cruelty

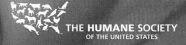

THE **HUMANE** SOCIETY
OF THE UNITED STATES

ZEN PALATE [v] **$$** 👍

Full service
Asian vegetarian
All major cards
No alcohol
www.zenpalate.com
See description under Midtown West

115 East 18th Street
brt/ Park Avenue/ Irving Place
212-387-8885
daily 11:30am-10:45pm

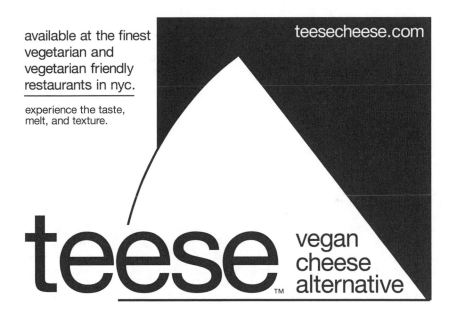

GOBO [ve]$$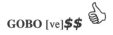

Full service	402 Sixth Avenue
Organic, Asian-Western fusion cuisine	at 8th Street
All cards	212-255-3242
Organic beer & wine	Su-We 11:30am-11:30pm
www.goborestaurant.com	Th-Sa 11:30am-12am

The atmosphere of Gobo-- the Japanese word for the root vegetable, burdock--is reminiscent of the tastefully decorated Zen Palate restaurants. The comparison is entirely appropriate because the owners of Gobo, Darryn and David Wu are the sons of the owners of Zen Palate, Mr. and Mrs. Tiehjyh Wu. Just as Zen Palate invokes the influence of Buddhism as their raison d' etre, so there is a statue of the Buddha prominently displayed at Gobo; he is smiling his blessing upon Gobo food, which is faithful to the Buddha's first precept of ahimsa (non-violence to all living creatures).

Gobo is proof of the fact that one can be a principled vegetarian yet enjoy the most exquisite food. For the food at Gobo's outstrips the cuisine of its parent restaurant Zen Palate. (This is ironic because most of the dishes were created by Mrs. Wu, the co-owner of Zen Palate). We started our dinner with a smoothie called The Awakening (mango, cherry and wolfberry), which was truly ambrosial. With our taste buds duly awakened, we were in a fit condition to enjoy the entrees, which were also very much to our taste--Sizzling Soy Cutlet Platter with Black Pepper Sauce, and the Soy Filet with Coconut Curry Rice. The desserts, all of which are vegan, were also extraordinary. We relished the Multi-layered Chocolate Cake and the Coconut-Chocolate Pudding with Mango Puree.

There are two non-vegan dishes--Avocado Tartare, which contains honey; and Crispy Spinach and Soy Cheese Wontons, which contains casein, a cows' milk extract, and egg, an ingredient in the won ton wrappers. Cow's milk, alas, is also available to tea and coffee drinkers who prefer it to the soy milk that is on offer.

The talk is that, if it is successful, Gobo plans to franchise the restaurant. Judging from the impeccable service, the attractive decor and the exquisite food, the burdock will soon be taking root in other American cities.

See other location under Upper East Side.

HUMMUS PLACE I [v]$

Full Service
Israeli vegetarian, kosher

99 Macdougal Street
bet. W. 3rd/ Bleecker Streets
212-533-3089

HUMMUS PLACE IV [v] $

Full Service
Israeli vegetarian, kosher
All cards
Wine & Beer

71 7th Avenue South
bet. Barrow/Bleecker Streets
212-924-2033
Su-Th 11am-12am
Fr-Sa 11am-2am

New York already has single-food-item restaurants dedicated to the French Fry, the Falafel, the Baked Potato, the Crepe, the Dosa, the Pancake, the Doughnut, Popcorn, Soup, and the Noodle; there is even a Candy bar (Dylan's)--so why not a restaurant devoted soley to Hummus? At Hummus Place, a tidy little beanery with walls the color of tahini, you can order two different styles of hummus--one made from fava beans and chickpeas, Hummus Foul (pronounced fool), and the other made from whole chickpeas, Hummus Masabacha. The fava beans and the chickpeas are imported from Israel to insure quality and freshness. The beans are then set to soak overnight and are chopped up in a huge Robotcoupe; then cooked for a full five hours. The hummus is served with a snow white tahini which is also imported from Israel.Two of the dishes are made with eggs; so vegans must tell the chef to hold the eggs!

Fittingly enough, the man who founded Hummus Place is an Israeli named Ori Apple, formerly of Kibbutz Maoz Haim. After his army service in Israel, Apple alighted in the Big Apple to study cooking at the French Culinary Institute in Soho. Having worked for a number of restaurants and a catering service in the city, Apple decided to strike out on his own. With the help and advice of his best friend--(now co-owner and chef of Hummus Place)--Nitzan Raz, Apple started Hummus Place. Apple's hummus is considered to be so authentic that Israelis joke that they no longer have any reason to visit Tel Aviv.

Because they've been cooked to a fare-thee-well-well, the flavor of the hummuses are a bit bland. Luckily, they come with a hot sauce on the side with a secret recipe whose base is cilantro. We found that the judicious seasoning of hummus with hot sauce enlivens the flavor and makes it go down much better. The hummus also comes with an Israeli Salad (whose ingredients are not imported from Israel). To give it an added fillip, we tried mixing the Israeli Salad in with the hummus and the hot sauce Then we used; the resultant mixture to fill a whole wheat pita pocket, which came with our order. This worked splendidly. We washed it all down with a cool glass of refreshing lemonade (also made with a secret recipe) that contains a sprig of fresh Israeli Mint. At the end of our meal, we left feeling satisfied and full of beans.

See other locations under East Village, MidTown West, and Upper West Side.

 Indicates we especially recommend this restaurant for the quality of the food.

INTEGRAL YOGA NATURAL FOODS [ve] $

Take-out counter
International
All cards
No alcohol
www. iynaturalfoods.com

229 West 13th Street
bet. 7th/ 8th Avenues
212-243-2642
M-F 8am-9:30pm
Sa 8am-8:30pm
Su 9am-8:30pm

Integral Yoga was started by Swami Satchidananda back in the seventies. The Swami taught that it was bad karma to consume or purvey animal flesh. Consequently, Integral Yoga is one of the few health food stores in the city that doesn't peddle flesh. Now you can tap into their good karma by having a meal there. Nestled into the North West corner of the store is one of the city's best vegan buffets. You may choose from such selections as Curried Black-Eyed Peas, Hot and Spicy Tofu and Bok Choy with Almonds. There is also a juice bar where you may purchase soups and veggie burgers. If you're a rawfoodist, take heart! There's a capacious salad bar; and in a refrigerated display case next to the buffet, there is an appetizing selection of raw vegetable pies, fruit pies, cakes, and cookies.

JIVAMUKTEA CAFE [ve] $$

Counter Service
Global vegan organic
All cards
No alcohol

841 Broadway (2nd Fl.)
bet. 13th/ 14th Streets
212-353-0214
M-F 11am-9pm
Sa-Su 1am-6pm

Overlooking the hubbub of Broadway in a spacious, airy setting, with an azure ceiling, antique chandeliers. and soaring stained glass windows, the new JivamukTea Café is housed inside the Jivamukti Yoga Center, which, from an ethical standpoint, is the best school of yoga in the city.

Unlike most yoga ashrams that give short shrift to *ahimsa,* which is the first precept of all classical yoga systems. it is clear that Jivamukti's founders, Sharon Gannon and David Life, uphold the view of Patanjali that if one is to advance spiritually in yoga one must eat non-violent food. In fact, in a recent interview, Sharon Gannon said," Veganism is essential to the practice of yoga, where you do not exploit animals for any purpose. Patanjali in the *Yoga Sutras,* gives *ahimsa* (non-harming of others) as the primary means to enlightenment." To that end, Sharon Gannon has created a menu that is conducive to attaining the higher states of yogic consciousness—and to having a transcendent dining experience.

This JivamukTea Café is figuratively a reincarnation of the first JivamukTea Cafe, which was managed by star chef Matthew Kenney, and went defunct not long after it opened. However, this new incarnation promises to have more staying power because it is that much better than its predecessor, which tried too hard to be trendy. This one's recipes come from co-founder Sharon Gannon's home kitchen, so they have a familial, home-style air to them.

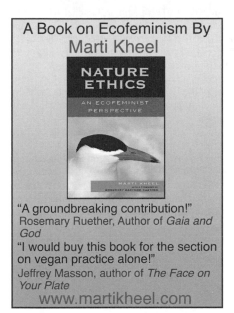
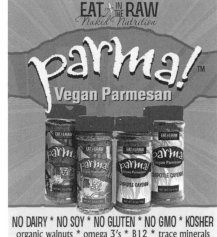
We tried their most popular sandwich, the Grilled Portobello Panino (portabella mushroom, sweet onions, nutritional yeast, chimchurri sauce on grilled sourdough). Yummy! Then we proceeded to have the Montana Salad, which contains seasonal vegetables, lettuce, cucumbers, black beans, quinoa, sprouts grown on the premises--all of it suffused with a turmeric-tahini dressing. Heavenly! To wash it down, we chugged a 3rd Eye Smoothie (acai, coconut water, banana, and organic vanilla extract). Ambrosial! For dessert, we had the Walnut Cake and the oversized Chocolate Chip Cookie that had just been plucked from the oven--with the result that the chips were still gooey and the dough was still soft and friable. Celestial! It was a vegan Toll House Cookie raised to a higher order of cookie. After dessert, as we watched the sunlight shimmering through the stained glass, we sipped, meditatively two generous cups of Love Blend Tea, a black tea with subtle chocolate overtones.

In spite of all the delicious food we had eaten, we seemed to float on air as we left the café, mumbling a *sotto voce* M-m-m-m-m mingled with Om-m-m-m-m-m.

NEW YORK DOSAS[ve]**$**

Food cart
South Indian
No cards
No alcohol

Washington Square Park
West 4th/ Sullivan Streets
917-710-2092
M-Sa 11am-4pm

We had to stand in line behind ten people to give our order to Thiru Kumar, the chef who works his magic at this outdoor food cart. Our order was for a Masala Dosa (a rolled rice-flour crepe stuffed with spicy potato mixture), Jafna Dosa (a rolled rice-flour crepe stuffed with Sambahl); Ponidicherry Utapam (a flat bread topped with fresh, chopped vegetables); and Iddly with Sambar (an Indian biscuit made from lentil flour and dipped in a spicy Sambar or soup).

Thiru, a native of Sri Lanka, works fast; he pours a batter made from crushed fermented rice and lentils on the griddle and within a few seconds, Utapam and Dosas appear, as if by magic. He fills them with spicy mashed potatoes and chopped fresh vegetables--and the result dosas and utapams worthy of the finest Indian restaurants.

Thiru packed our order into boxes; then we sat on a bench in Washington Square park and savored every morsel.

It's hard to believe that so much food can pour forth from one little food cart! In addition to the Dosas, one may order Samosas with vegetable fillings; Medhu Vada (lentil donuts), and the aforementioned Iddly with Sambar. Thiru also offers up a unique array of tinned fruit juices imported from Thailand--such as Rambutan juice, Longan juice, and, our favorite, Lychee juice-- that are available nowhere else in the city. Unusual for an Indian food establishment, vegans may dine here without having to ask about objectionable ingredients--as all the food is 100 per cent vegan. [Thiru bowed to pressure from vegan students at the NYU Vegan Society to make his food cart exclusively vegan. Now he himself has turned vegan.]

ORGANIC AVENUE-2 [ve] $$

Self service   43 8th Avenue
Organic raw food bar/boutique   bet. Jane/ /Horatio Streets
All major cards   212-358-0500
No alcohol   daily 8am-8pm
www.organicavenue.com

See description under SOHO.

OTARIAN [v] $

Counter service   154 Bleecker Street
Global ovo-lacto vegetarian   bet. Laguardia/Thompson Streets
All cards   212-614-6834
                                                          daily 11am-11pm

See description under Midtown West

RED BAMBOO [ve] *$$* 👍

	140 West 4th Street
Full service	bet. 6th/MacDougal
Asian soul food fusion	212-260-1212
All cards	M-F 12:30pm-12am
No alcohol	Sa-Su 12pm-12am
www.redbamboo-nyc.com	

"Soul Food with Asian overtones" is how the proprietor, Philip Wong, describes the cuisine At play here are multi-ethnic flavors such as Chinese, Korean, Thai, Indian. Creole and Soul Food. In most instances, the fusion of flavors works.

For appetizers, we had the Caribean Jerk Spiced Seitan, which was tangy and tasty, as were the Collard Green Rolls, the Popcorn Shrimp, and the gluten "pork" in the Tonkatsu Chops. We also sampled the Mango Chicken. and the Barbecue Buffalo Wings, which were finger lickin' good. However, on the debit side, the Seoul Pancake was too mushy and the sweet corn mashed potatoes were way too bland. We capped it all off with a scrumptious Death By Chocolate cake served with a dollop of vegan Mint Chocolate Chip ice-cream. The waiters were attentive and hovering.

The only difficulty that vegans might have with eating at Red Bamboo is that the menu is so unrelievedly mock-carnivorous that the mere sight of dishes with names like Satay Chicken, Popcorn Shrimp, and Roast Beef Sandwich, no matter how mock, might conjure unpleasant associations with the real thing. Nonetheless, Red Bamboo is a great place to take your meat-eating friends to show them how animal flesh may be mocked to perfection. Two dishes contain dairy and these are noted on the menu.

SACRED CHOW [v]*$$* 👍

	227 Sullivan Street
Full service	bet. West 3rd & Bleecker Streets
International & bakery	212-337-0863
V, AE, MC	M-F 9 am--11pm
Organic beer & wine	Sa-Su 11:30am-11pm
www.sacredchow.com	

Cliff Preefer, the owner of Sacred Chow used to be the head chef as well as the pastry chef, at Candle Cafe back in the mid-90's. Then he decided to strike out on his own and start a veg. delicatessen, which eventually gave place to this new restaurant of the same name. Casting about for a name for his eatery, he hit upon the inspired pun--"sacred chow." With its logo of the meditating cow, and its pun on sacred cow, could Cliff's restaurant have been anything but vegan? Unfortunately, yes. Cliff does serve dairy products in the shape of ice-cream and creamers for coffee. This is rather a desecration of that poor sacred cow, who is exploited for its exudate, is it not?

Apart from this notable lapse, there is an admirable respect for the cow that pervades the restaurant and its menu. There are usually about thirty vegan tapas on offer. The ones we sampled were extraordinary--Korean Tofu Cutlets, the Shredded Tofu Spa Salad, and Curried Steamed Broccoli. The Hero Sandwich that we had as a main course --Roasted Black Olive Seitan, with molten vegan Mozzarella --was so good that we had to stifle a shout of jubilation. [Fact is: Cliff's Hero sandwiches and pastries are so sought-after that he retails them to other snackeries around the city--like the one in the cafe at the Angelika Cinema.]

While we munched our Heroes, amid the warm, rouge tints of the interior decor, we sipped one of Cliff's frozen smoothies, which he calls Gym Body (bananas, toasted almonds, cinnamon, flax oil and apple juice). This was so satisfying that we could easily have made a meal of it.

For dessert we inhaled Cliff's famous Velvet Triple Chocolate Brownie with a side scoop of organic vegan Raspberry Ice-Cream. Cliff, [excuse the bad pun], we will be dropping over quite often, (especially if S. C. becomes 100% vegan).

• On a recent visit, [2012] we were delighted to learn that Sacred Chow has gone completely vegan! Did our caustic review have anything to do with their eliminating the mammary secretions from their meun? We fervently hope so! Kudos to Cliff.

SOY & SAKE [v] $$

Full service	47-49 Seventh Avenue South
Japanese-pan Asian	bet.Bleecker / Morton Streets
All Cards	212-255-2848
Sake bar	M-Sa 9am-9pm
www.soyandsaake.com	

Another first for New York: Soy 'N' Sake is New York'--if not the world's--first vegetarian sushi bar. Commonly, sushi contains fish; however, in this sushi bar, the sushi rolls are blessedly fin-, feather- and flesh-free. The place is owned by the same family who gave us those other landmarks of vegetarian gastronomy: VP-2 (Chinese} and Red Bamboo.(a fusion of pan-Asian and Southern Soul).

Seated comfortably at a table that looked onto 7th Avenue South, we started with the Mock Tuna (a rice wrapper enrobes avocado and marinated mock tuna chunks); We then had a Lettuce Wrap (a tender leaf of lettuce wraps a mixture of string beans, jicamas, carrots, grilled tofu, and rice-noodles served with a side of vegan hoisin sauce). The portions were so generous and so artfully prepared that we felt fully satisfied after downing the wrap and roll. Consequently, we decided to call it an evening after sharing one more sushi roll—the Hawaiian Roll (a sweetish tasting combination of banana chunks and Asian pear. enrobed in a wrapper of thin rice dough, and sliced into thin rounds).

Before leaving, we cast a wistful glance at the menu, feeling a pang of regret that we would never be able to taste any of the other delectable dishes. Towards the end of the meal, we had got up to explore the interior of the restaurant when we noticed something that troubled us deeply, and made us vow that as ethical vegans we could not, in good conscience, return to eat h ere. The full bar--where a variety of sakes and other alcoholic drinks are dispensed--is walled off by a floor-to-ceiling aquarium. It is painfully ironic that while the sushi contains no fish, the aquarium in the sushi bar not only contains fish, but exploits them for gaudy visual effects

'sNICE [v] $

Self service
Sandwiches, salads, baked goods
All cards
Beer & wine

45 8th Avenue
at 4th Street
212-645-0310
daily 7:30am-10pm

'sWonderful, 'sMarvelous, 'sNice? You'll surely agree that this coffee shop-cum-bistro deserves a loftier superlative than merely nice. Really, the food is nothing short of 'sMarvelous! That was our original evaluation of 'sNice during the first three years of its existence. Now, we're chagrined to report that, we've detected a dropoff in quality, which seems to have coincided with sNice's expansion into Park Slope, Brooklyn. Gone are the board games, children's toys, the Fizzi waters, and the vivid-tasting wraps that we used to adore. We've taken a number of our friends there over the past year. To a person, they've complained that the smoothies, the wraps and the clumps of salad served with them are insipid-tasting and monotonous. "The wraps smack of a doughy blandness with a sameness of flavor," said they. We are reluctantly forced to concur. Perhaps most off-putting of all, though, is the owner's attitude towards veganism, which is one of thinly disguised hostility. When asked if he would ever remove the honey, milk, Brie Cheese, Cream Cheese, Gorgonzola Cheese, Bleu Cheese, Goat Cheese, Mozzarella Cheese, Swiss Cheese, Parmesan Cheese, [Hey! Eight varieties of cheese on the menu! Is this a veg. bistro or a cheese shop?] and other mammary secretions from his menu, he bristled with indignation, and said "Never!"

'sOkay, 'sBland, 'sCheesy, but not 'sMarvelous, as it used to be. Let's hope that he may return to his former high standards, and go vegan!

See other locations under Greenwich Village and Brooklyn.

TAIM [v] $
Counter service
Kosher Israeli falafel shack
All cards
No alcohol
www.taimnyc.com

222 Waverly Place
at 7th Avenue
212-691-1287
M-Su 11am-10:30pm

According to our researches, the first bona fide vegetarian Israeli falafel shack in NYC is this diminutive Greenwich Village spot called Taim. Since it was opened by Einat Admony, Taim's lady chef, two years ago, a number of others have sprung up, apparently, in imitation. Hummus

Place on MacDougal Street and Moaz on Union Square East. Curiously enough, none of the owners of these ovo-lacto vegetarian falafel shacks is a vegetarian. They purvey vegetarian food simply because it is more expedient, more healthful, and hygienic to do so.

"Taim," which means delicious in Hebrew, is aptly named. "Taim" was practically every dish we tried here. We particularly relished the Falafel Sandwich. A pita pocket was filled with our choice of Green, Red or Harissa falafel balls and presented to us with side dishes of Israeli salad, pickled green cabbage, and tahini. The pickled carrot and beet salads were pleasingly tart and tasty. We also savored the Sabich (a pita sandwich of fried eggplant, slathered with pickles, onions, tahini and two types of hot sauce. The Sabich was invented by the Lord Sandwich of Israel-- Oved, a one-name-only denizen of the Tel Aviv suburb, Givatayim. It has since become the most popular hand-held food item in Israel. However, before ordering the Sabich, it is important to tell the chef to hold the eggs, because for some strange reason, a chick embryo is felt to be an obligatory ingredient in this dish.

We really liked their home-made French fries that we would rank second only to those of Freedom Tripodi of FoodSwings in Williamsburg. We tossed off a delicious Strawberry-Raspberry-Thai-Basil smoothie, and a Ginger-Mint lemonade, which could make this place one of the city's better juice bars, were it not drenched in milk. However, they use whole and skim milk in their smoothies, so vegans should ask that the blender be washed, before making a non-dairy smoothie, to expel any caseous residues/ The service staff will honor your request with alacrity.

VEGETARIAN'S PARADISE-2 *$$* 🖐

Full service
Chinese
$4.95-12.95 (AE,MC,V)
No alcohol

140 / 144 West 4th Street
bet. Sixth Ave/ MacDougal Street
212-260-7130/7141
M-Th 12pm-11pm, F-Sa 12pm-12am

We know, you've long since given up ordering Peking Spare Ribs, Sweet and Pungent Pork and Squid in Black Bean Sauce. Do it anyway. The meaty names just help identify traditional Chinese dishes that VP's Buddhist chefs prepare exclusively without animal products (using soy, wheat, and arrowroot substitutes). The food is authentic and reasonably priced, served in a modern, sleek restaurant . One of the best of this type of place.

🖐 Indicates we especially recommend this restaurant for the quality of the food

EAST VILLAGE
(Houston to East 14th Street, Fifth Avenue to the East River)

ANGELICA KITCHEN [ve] $$ 🖒

Full service
Natural
No cards
No alcohol

300 E 12th Street
at Second Avenue
212-228-2909
daily 11:30am-10:30pm

Hands down one of the best vegan restaurants anywhere. For 25 years Angelica Kitchen has set the standard for fresh organic fare with a conscience.

Each day there are two very special, always new, special entrees such as "Here Today--Gone Tamale'" (Festive tamales made with Iroquois white corn masa and roasted home-made seitan, chipotle and ancho chili peppers, all wrapped in a corn husk served with tomato-cilantro salsa, over a baby lima bean sauce, with baby lettuces and steamed local asparagus). Or try the norimake rolls with grilled tempeh, home-made pickled carrots and brown rice; like sushi, they're rolled in nori seaweed .

For those who wish to try Angelica Kitchen's tasty dishes at home, the Angelica Home Kitchen Cookbook by Leslie McEachern (the owner) is for sale in the restaurant. It includes over 100 recipes from the menu archives that have been specially formulated for the home cook. The book also sets forth Leslie's philosophy and principles for running a socially conscious business, and it features profiles of the farmers and artisans who provide the restaurant with the ingredients for their delicious fare.

Angelica's is a dessertatarian's delight. We swooned over the rhubarb layer cake with strawberry frosting and the coconut flan with pineapple salsa was unforgettable. Consistently fresh, flavorful and satisfying, the whole vital menu proves why the outstanding reputation of Angelica Kitchen is so richly deserved Take-out next door.

BLOSSOM DU JOUR- SPORTS CAFE[ve] $$ 🖒

Counter Service
Vegan organic fast ;food.
Visa, Master Card
No alcohol
www. Blossomdujour.com

62 Cooper Square
Inside NHYRC (open to the public)
212-228-1659
M-F 8am-10pm
Sa-Su 10am-10pm

See Description Under Midtown West and other location under Upper West Side.

CAFE VIVA [A.K.A. VIVA HERBAL PIZZERIA] [v] $

Counter service
Italian, organic, kosher
All cards
No alcohol

179 Second Avenue
bet. 11th / 12th Streets
212-420-8801
daily 11am-11pm
Sa-Su 11am-12am

See /Description under Upper West Side

CARAVAN OF DREAMS [ve] $$$ 👍

Full service
International organic, kosher
V,MC
Full bar, organic beer & wine
www.caravanofdreams.net/

405 East 6th Street
bet. First Ave/Avenue A
212-254-1613
M,Su 11am-11pm, Sa 11am-12am
Sa,,Su brunch 11am-5pm

Organic vegetarian food in a hippy atmosphere of long hair, mix and match furniture and live music almost every night. Quite relaxing during non-peak hours. No dairy is used; a few years ago, Caravan went completely vegan. Black bean chili, grilled polenta, African spinach stew over rice, pasta, burritos, quesadilla, wild rice and cremini risotto croquettes, large salads, sandwiches, "greens of the day." A pleasure. Recently Caravan has begun serving raw-food entrees every day. It also serves a range of raw soups and desserts. Their avocado coconut soup is simply ravishing! And their raw raspberry cake bears comparison with any baked cake in town. Every night, their new raw chef creates live food specials that rotate every week. We enjoyed the Taco Salad, the Live Mock Meat Balls, the Live Nachos, and the Live Sandwich. Obviously Caravan's Dreams have come to life.

CURLY'S VEGETARIAN LUNCH [v] $$

Full Service
American fast food
All cards
Beer & Sangria

328 East 14th Street
bet. 1st & 2nd Avenues
212-598-9998
Daily 11am-11pm

Rectangular in shape, with cream-colored walls, decorated with two parallel mango stripes, and a lozenge-shaped mirror, there is nothing kinky about Curly's Vegetarian Lunch--except the curly French fries-and the Cubano Sandwich. They have a kinky flavor that wraps itself around your tongue and won't let go. As a rule, we don't care much for mock meat--it's too rereminiscent of the real thing--but we're making an exception for Curly's Cubano. Heaven help the folks who eat the real (carnivorous) Cubano: it has enough cholesterol to thrombose a regiment of Visigoths.

But Curly's vegan Cubano with its mock ham, mock dark meat, mock cheese, sans casein, and pickle has a raffish appeal to the taste buds that is not to be denied. Ditto for the mock Buffalo wings. Both by the way are "two-hanky" specials that require two or more napkins to eat without spotting one's blouse. We also savored the Cashew Sofrito (Unsalted cashew nuts in a sofrito of tomato, peppers, olives and achiote. served over fried plantain with back beans and grain). And you don't have to go anywhere else for dessert. Curly's serves a full complement of Vegan Treats' pies and cakes that Veg-City Diner was famous for.

Curly's Vegetarian Lunch seems a quirky name for a restaurant. But a glance at the back page of the menu explains everything. There, the founders and owners of Curly's--David and Jean--have thoughtfully provided the story of how the restaurant got its name. Curly, the grandfather of David, owned a diner in New Hampshire. After a catastrophic flood washed away most of the town, Curly provided free food for the townspeople, and became a local hero. David, wanted to pay tribute to his grandfather's food as well as his unsung heroism.

We almost forgot to mention that Curly's is the brainchild of David and his wife Jean, the former owners of the late-lamented Veg-City Diner, which was forced to close because of a freak kitchen fire. Neither David nor his wife is a vegetarian, but they love to prepare vegetarian food, and delight in inventing new ways to use mock meats. David is also the former owner of urritoville, the only Mexican restaurant in New York City that has vegan sour cream; he has an abiding love affair with Mexican cuisine. His contract with the buyers of Buttitoville won't let him make Mexican food at Curly's. His vegan Cubano is an homage to the Vegan Mexican cuisine of his heart's desire. Someday, he promises to open a 100 per cent vegan Mexican restaurant. On that day, we'll be the first in line.

DIRT CANDY $$$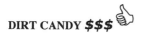

Full service
Vegetarian haute cuisine
All major cards
Wine
www.dirtcandynyc.com

430 East 9th Street
bet. First/ A Avenues
212-228-7732
T-Sa 5:30pm-11pm

Casting about for a euphemistic name for her restaurant that didn't feature the highly charged "V" word, Amanda Cohen, the owner-chef, hit upon "Dirt Candy." as a synonym for vegetables. At the foot of her menu, she has written this epigraph: "Made of little more than water and sunlight, vegetables are candy from the dirt. We want you to relax, have fun and be surprised at how good they can be."

The food is ovo-lacto vegetarian; so it's mandatory for vegans to declare themselves at the start of the meal or, preferably, when making reservations. Reservations are a must because the room holds only 19 diners who sit cheek by jowl. Crammed into this same small room, is a mini-bathroom and a tmicro-kitchen where food is prepared, orders are plated, and dishes are washed and dried.

Despite the close quarters, Dirt Candy is a fitting showcase for Amanda's talents, not only as a creative chef but also as a restaurant manager. She doesn't just stir the pot and point a spatula at uniformed flunkies; she waits on tables, she cooks, and she even washes dishes in a hyperkinetic blur of energy that is as enthralling to watch as the food is to eat.

Such an air of *bonhommie* pervades the room that we chatted amiably with the diners to our left and right, as if we were all seated at a communal table. Topic A was the food and how *exquise* it was. Each course evoked oooh's and aaah's. We started with peppery Jalapeno Hush Puppies which were served with an ambrosial tasting maple vegan spread. For teetotalers, like us, the waitress poured an endless flow of non-alcoholic Riesling wine [Navarro Vineyards] from California. Next, we had the Mixed Green Salad with mock cheese croutons and Candied Grapefruit Pops. For the main course, we had The Crispy Tofu in Green Ragout, which consisted of grilled tofu topped with a bundle of micro-greens and a-swim in a sauce made from chopped Brussels sprouts and vivid, crunchy vegetables. Having cheffed at rawfoods restaurants like Pure Food and Wine under Matthew "Everyday Raw" Kenney, Amanda, has gained the insight that vegetables are more flavorful and colorful when they are slightly undercooked. For dessert, Amanda served us a layered vegan ice cream bar that--taken with all the other wondrous dishes of Amanda's devising--has given us a permanent sweet tooth for Dirt Candy

HUMMUS PLACE II [v] $

Full Service
Israeli vegetarian, kosher
All cards
Wine & Beer

109 St. Marks Place
bet. 1st & A Avenues
212-529-9198
Su-Th 11am-12am
Fr-Sa 11am-2am

See description under Greenwich Village, and other location under Upper West Side.

JUICE PRESS-2 , THE [ve] $$

Counter service
Organic Juices and raw food
All Cards
No alcohol

279 East 10th Street
bet. 1st /A Avenues/
212-777-0034
darily 8am-8pm

JUICE PRESS, THE [ve] $$

Counter service
Organic Juices and raw food
All Cards
No alcohol
Thejuicepressonline.com

70 East 1st Street
bet. 1st / 2nd Avenues/
212-777-0034
darily 8am-8pm

When he was a much younger man, Marcus Antebi, the founder of The Juice Press, worked with his father in the antiques business. Ironically enough, now that he is approaching middle age, he's in the rejuvenation business. He takes prematurely antique and wizened younger folk, and by putting them on a vegan raw food diet--interspersed with juice cleanses--he reinvigorates them in body as well as in spirit

With the muscular physique and the high verve of the Muay Thai kick-boxer that he is, Marcus is the best advertisement for his vegan rawfoodist lifestyle. Recently a reporter from the New York Times Style section put herself under Marcus's tutelage and afterwards felt transfigured. On Day 10 of her program, she was ecstatic over losing 11 pounds. and has become a confessed addict of the vegan raw foods and juice elixirs that helped her shed her surplus poundage—such as "Complete Source"(carrot, celery, spinach, parsley). The juice blends, are hydraulically expressed from organic fruits and vegetables by powerful Norwalk Juicers,. [Norwalk Juicers--the most efficient juicers on the market—are used because they minimize nutrient and enzyme loss.]

Ideally, Marcus tells us, the juice cleanses are a preparation for embarking on a high raw vegan diet. Marcus's mentor, Dr. Fred Bisci , who is in his early 80s , but could pass for a youthful 50, has been extolling the virtues of a raw food vegan diet for more than 40 years. His motto is "It's not what you put into your body, but what you leave out."

What we put into our body, however, was not only delicious, but also energizing and uplifting. Which is seldom one's condition after a cooked meal. It's important to emphasize that, despite its name, The Juice Press, serves up some of the tastiest and most healthful solid food in town. We started with the Marinated Kale Salad (marinated kale, steeped in a lime dressing, and nutritional yeast is topped with nori, tomato, avocado, and sprouts.) Next we had their Ravioli (raw sliced turnips are filled with homemade vegan cashew cheese, garnished with black sesame seeds, and served with homemade raw pesto.) For dessert, we ate their raw Acai Nut Mix (raw organic acai berry, buckwheat, sunflower, walnuts, flax, almonds, coconut oil, vanilla, cacao, blueberry).

The Juice Press is so successful that it has already expanded to three branches within the space of a year. Rawfoodism and Norwalk cold pressed juices seem to be riding the crest of a wave that is engulfing (and cleansing) the city.

KAJITSU $$$$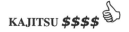

Full service
Japanese vegan haute cuisine
All major cards
Beer & sake
www.kajitsunyc.com

414 East 9th Street
bet. First/ A Avenues
212-228-4873
T-Su 5:30pm-10pm

The food served at Kajitsu is pure *shojin ryori* or vegan food, which originated in the Buddhist temples of Japan. The dining area has the stark simplicity of a Kyoto temple, with geometric lines and light dappled wood surfaces. There are two menus: One is a four-course $50 one. The other is an eight-course $70 one. Except for the Housemade Soba Noodles, which are a constant, the menus change monthly and feature food items that look penitential and austere, but in the hands of chef Masato Nishihara, are transformed into dishes that are interesting and flavorful, albeit a touch too salty for our taste.

We opted for the more expensive menu and were regaled with such dishes as Agar Agar Aspic with Summer Vegetables Served with Umami Soy Sauce. (Liliputian summer vegetables

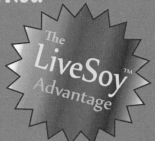
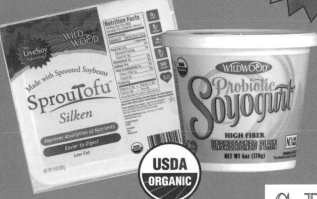
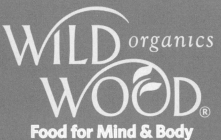

We opted for the more expensive menu and were regaled with such dishes as Agar Agar Aspic with Summer Vegetables Served with Umami Soy Sauce. (Liliputian summer vegetables were suspended in a tasty soy-sauce-soaked gelatinous goo.) This was followed by a hearty Celery Root Soup that was flavored with red daikon and kohlrabi. We especially liked the next courses-- poached tomatoes, the tempura vegetables and the corn croquettes. The dominant flavor note in all the dishes is saltiness, Even the dessert--Sweetened Edamame Mochi with Pistachio Nuts-- smacked of salt.

The owners of Kajitsu are emphatically not vegan and in fact are aiming to attract food snobs and gastronomes. This is reflected in the price of the food, which is more redolent of the temples of commerce than of the Zen temples of Kyoto. Our bill at the end of the meal came to more than $200 including tax and tip. Eating at Kajitsu then is an exercise in conspicuous consumption. Perhaps this is not a bad thing. Veganism will advance socially only when it is invested with snob appeal.

KATE'S JOINT [v] $$

	58 Avenue B
Full Service	bet. 4th / 5th Streets
American faux fifties diner style	212-777-7059
AE, MC,V	Su-Th 9 am-12am
Beer & wine	F-Sa 9am-2am

Eating at Kate's Joint is like stepping into a Norman Rockwell painting from the fifties. The food as well as the atmosphere are faux fifties--a time when restaurants were called "joints", coffee was called "java," and music poured from the juke box. The food, unlike the food of the fifties, is healthy vegan and vegetarian. Some of the dishes are take-offs on the diner food of the fifties that tasted so good, but was so bad for you. Dishes like Fake Steak, Mock Shepherd's Pie with Salad, Southern Fried Tofu, and Apple Crumb Cake conjure up the fifties originals without inducing a coronary on the way home. [Vegans should be cautious when ordering any dish that contain mock cheese; they may contain casein. Ask the chef.] This is a great place to take your non-veg. friends to coax them off meat, but it's a positive pleasure for anyone. As a chef Kate is great. She and her sister do all the cooking and baking on the premises. Their American home-style dishes are highly original and very tasty. In keeping with the trend towards rawfood eating among vegans and vegetarians, Kate is now offering an organic living-foods menu.

KENOSHA [v] $

	543 East Twelfth Street
Counter service	bet. Avenues A/ B
Midwestern American & South Indian	212-945-8053
No cards	daily 11am-11pm
No alcohol	

Kenosha is the name of a small town in Wisconsin, which is famous for being the birthplace of the great film director and actor Orson Welles. It's also noted for being the cradle for radio announcers, who were recruited for the country's airwaves because they grew up speaking unaccented Midwestern English. So what's a nice town like Kenosha doing in a place like this? Well, one of the owners is from Kenosha, and he was nostalgic for his hometown. The other owner is Kumi Kulantri of Mumbai, the Indian restaurateur, who has had at least half a dozen restaurants--Dosaria, Thali, Tiffin, et al., shot out from under him. Together they form one of the New York restaurant scene's oddest couples. Their fare is a combination of Midwestern America meets upper middle class Mumbai. We tried their Mango Soup, which is really, really good, and their Veggie Burgers, which were made with colorful shredded vegetables. Kumi made us some delicious Soy Milk Mango Lassis for dessert. We told them that to complete the decor they should put some pictures of Orson Welles on the wall.

•As of this writing, 2012, we are waiting impatiently for Kumi to open Kenosha.

LAN CAFE [v] $ 👍

Full service	342 East 6th Street
Vietnamese	bet. 1st/ 2nd Avenue
Cash only	212-228-8325
Beer & wine	Tu-Su 2pm-11pm

Last summer, we sampled vegan dishes in some Vietnamese restaurants in Hawaii--where there is a large settlement of Vietnamese folk, but, alas, no vegan Vietnamese restaurants. Admittedly, the food was very good, but the food at Lan Cafe--New York's first vegan Vietnamese restaurant--surpasses that of the best in Honolulu. Perhaps it's because the co-owner/chef --Cao Ky and his wife Lan--are devout Mahayana Buddhists and therefore are ethical vegans. Hence, the food is 100% cruelty-free , and, on our many visits, the pure, unalloyed flavors of this essentially Buddhist Vietnamese cuisine shone forth.

`   In fact, the food at Lan Cafe is so exquisite, that we played a little parlor game--we challenged each other to find a dish on the menu that we didn't like. After repeated visits, we exhausted the menu without being able to find a dish that we didn't adore. All are extraordinary. At Lan Cafe, we must speak of the extraordinary among extraordinaries. These are the best vegan eats of the East!

We recommend that you start with the classic Vietnamese dish --a staple on the menus of restaurants in Saigon--Green Papaya Salad with Mock Shrimp. Follow this with Pho--another classic Vietnamese dish. A capacious bowl is filled with a healthy serving of vegetable broth aswim with long rice noodles, and vegetarian beef. On the side are served bean sprouts and basil leaves. At intervals, these are to be added to the Pho. The flavors, of both the Green Papaya Salad and the Pho, were stupendous!

Fact is: Frank, the manager, had warned us that the Pho at Lan Cafe is so filling that there is scant room for anything else. He was right. We wanted to try the Curried Lemon Grass Seitan, and the Baguettes with Vegetarian Sausage and the one with Vegetarian Mock Ham (an incongruous Gallicism here that is doubtless the legacy of the French colonial occupation of Vietnam, as is the name of that glorious soup, pho, which is a corruption of the French word for fire *feu*.)--but we had to postpone those gustatory sensations for our next visit. Our only puzzlement was why was it so easy to find a table here? By rights, there should be lines of vegan gourmets winding around the block.

How did the Lan Cafe get its name. In Vietnamese the word "lan" means "orchid." "Orchidaceous" would aptly describe the cuisine--exotic, eye-filling, and drop-dead delicious!

LULA"S SWEET APOTHECARY [ve] $

	516 East 6th Street
Counter service	bet. Avenues A & B
Gourmet vegan ice-cream	646-912-4549
No cards	Su, Tu, W 3pm-10pm
No alcohol	Th,F, Sa 3pm-11:30pm
www.lulasweet.com	

Derek and Blythe, are the owners of New York's first vegan ice-cream parlor. They earned their stripes in Philadelphia where for two years they operated a food truck called Viva Las Vegans on the campus of Drexel University. While plying their trade on the Drexel campus, they conceived the bright idea of opening a vegan ice-cream parlor in NYC. Undaunted, they sold Viva Las Vegans; moved to New York City; and, in October, 2008, opened Lula's which is named for Blythe's niece. The rest is vegan history, or should we say her-story?

Half-Vietnamese, and all-American, Blythe is an alumna of the elite Mt. Holyoke College in Massachusetts. Her business partner, Derek, is from Ireland and speaks with an engaging brogue. An indefatigable worker, with the skills (and muscles) of a cabinet-maker, Derek built the oak paneled interior that recalls an old-time ice-cream parlor, vintage 1947.

Think of Lula's then as an old-fashioned drugstore-cum-soda fountain without the drugstore, (and the drugstore cowboys). It evokes the sort of place that gave us the term "soda jerk" and; and where Pemberton invented the recipe for Coca-Cola; and where movie stars like Lana Turner were "discovered." It displays apothecary jars stuffed with sweets, and dispenses all the old soda-fountain treats--eggless egg-creams, banana splits, and. of course, the immortal sundae.

The ice-creams are nut-, water-, and soy-based of which a high preponderance are nut-based. Last time we were there, Blythe and Derek--who are constantly experimenting with new flavors-- had just contrived chocolate malt and vanilla malt flavors; they were so delicious that we hope they'll become staples. Some of our other favorites include coconut fudge; peanut-butter fudge; cake-batter soft serve twist; and cinnamon-pecan.

MAOZ III [v] $

Counter service	59 East 8th Street
Israeli falafel shack, kosher	bet. Broadway/ University Place
All Cards	212-420-5999
No alcohol	daily 11am-12am
www.maozusa.com	

See description under Midtown East and other location under Upper West Side.

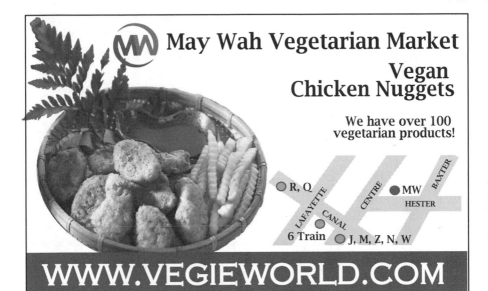
POMMES FRITES [v] $

Counter Service
Belgian French fries
No cards
No alcohol

123 Second Avenue
bet. Seventh/ Eighth Streets
212-674-1234
daily 11:30am-Midnight

Studies have shown that people go to burger joints mainly for the French fries. With the opening of Pommes Frites and its opposite number, B. Frites at 1657 Broadway, it's now possible for vegetarians to dine on French Fries without having to make a clandestine visit to the Golden Arches. In Belgium, the *maison de pommes frites* is a thriving concern. So some enterprising Americans have imported the idea to New York and judging from the lines that form up at Pommes Frites and B. Frites, it's really taking hold. The fries at Pommes Frites are double cooked in the Belgian manner, and are served with a range of tasty sauces. For vegans, it's necessary to inquire about the composition of the sauces as some may contain mayonnaise and other objectionable ingredients. We managed quite nicely with a double cone of fries that we dipped alternately in etchup and mustard, which are on the house; the other sauces are fifty cents extra.

PUKK [v] $$

Full service
Thai vegetarian
All cards
Beer, wine, champagne
www.pukknyc.com

75 First Avenue
bet. 4th/ 5th Streets
212-253-2741
daily 11:30am-11pm

A four-letter word in Thai that means "vegetable," Pukk is an apt name for this all-vegetarian Thai restaurant. Imaginatively designed to make maximum use of the rather cramped dining spaces, Pukk is a model of elegant compression. But the menu enables one to dine spaciously on delicious Thai vegetarian fare. It's not quite vegan here because, inexplicably they serve eggs?!!!? So vegans should inquire about eggs in the noodles, in the pastries, in the soups, and sauces, etc. But everything else is impeccably plant-based. In fact, the Pukksters thoughtfully provide soy milk for tea, coffee, and smoothies. For starters, try the Tom Yum Soup, a yummy soup that is aswim with chunks of spiced tofu, mushrooms, scallions and cilantro; then try the Curry Thai Pancake, a flaky crepe served in a piquant curry sauce. Follow this with the Faux Salmon; or, if you prefer to avoid faux meats, try the tofu dishes--such as Stuffed Tofu, or the Son-in-Law Tofu--at which Thai chefs excel. If there is a rawfooder in your midst, then he or she will be certain to enjoy the All Green Salad, which layers fresh vegetables on a mound of fresh greens. It is nattily and nuttily dressed with a splash of spicy peanut sauce.

    Dessert here is a bit of an anticlimax after the crescendo of flavors leading up to it. So we recommend ambling over to Caravan of Dreams, or Babycakes for a truly scrumptious dessert. Although the food here is not so good as that of the Thai vegan restaurant in Montreal called Chu Chai, which for our money is one of the best vegan restaurant in the world, it is good enough, because of its sheer exoticism, to be one of the better vegetarian restaurants in New York

QUINTESSENCE [ve] $$$

Full Service
Raw food vegetarian
All cards
No alcohol
www.raw-q.com

263 East 10th Street
bet. 1st Avenue/ Avenue A
646-654-1823
daily 11:am-11pm

For skeptics who think that raw food is a penitential diet of roots, shoots and fruits, Tolentin and her business partner Dan Hoyt, who have been strict rawfoodists for four years, are on a mission to show people that rawfood can be as toothsome as it is nutritious. So admirably have they succeeded that you'd swear that some of the dishes are cooked. Ironically, the mark of a good raw food dish is that it tastes as if it's been cooked. This is certainly true of the Sun Burger, a hearty patty made of sunflower and flaxseed meal mixed with chopped celery, onions, red pepper and herbs dehydrated to a burger consistency and served between slices of dehydrated bread. {The temperature of the dehydrator in which the breads are baked must never rise above an enzyme-killing 120 degrees). Another entree, the Caribbean Nut Meatballs which are served in an aromatic, zesty pineapple-tomato sauce also earns the accolade: "Tastes as if it's been

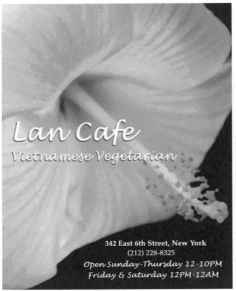
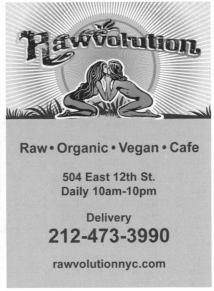
cooked." The Coconut Cream Pie and the Pecan Pie are the quintessence of desserts, fired or unfired, anywhere in the city.

• We were gratified to learn that Quintessence is now 100 percent organic and vegan. When they first opened, we lobbied for them to stop using honey in their dishes, and we like to think that we have played a small role in their going completely vegan. Credit to chef Dan!

RAWVOLUTION [ve] $$ 👍

Counter service
Raw, organic, vegan cafe
All cards
No alcohol
www.rawvolutionnyc.com

504 East 12th Street
bet. A / B Avenues
212-473-3990
daily 10am-10-pm

Recently Janabai Amsden, the co-owner of RAWvolution, was the subject of a feature article in the WSJ, titled Raw Food is Penetrating Deeper into NYC. She and her restaurant, RAWvolution, were the focus of the article because RAWvolution is emblematic of the higher standards and higher tastes that have taken root in the vegan raw food movement. Fact is, Janabai, the former head raw food chef at the Essene retreat, Tree of Life in Arizona, and her husband Matt, author of the eponymous bestselling raw prep book, RAWvolution, have spearheaded RAW, an acronym that stands for Raw Alliance Worldwide, which seeks to set standards for the preparation of raw food. RAWvolution, the restaurant, is a case in point. It exemplifies the highest standards in vegan raw food preparation and taste.

In a marriage made in Raw Heaven, Janabai and Matt married in 2005. Janabai and Matt had met in LA where Janabai ran a raw food boutique, called Euphoria. They started selling Matt's boxed living foods meals out of Euphoria. When the orders came flooding in, they opened a stand alone restaurant called Euphoria Loves RAWvolution Cafe. Appropriately enough: out of Euphoria came the RAWvolution!

In Santa Monica, (where it originated), Euphoria Loves RAWvolution Café does such a thriving business that they decided to open a branch on the East Coast, *i.e.*, the East Village of NYC, affectionately known as "raw vegan central." We are the lucky beneficiaries of that decision.

We started with a Tomato and "Cheese" Bagel Sandwich with the " cream cheese" having been made from cashew cheese. The raw bagel was made from zucchini and almond pulp; then dehydrated in a dehydrator. It was extraordinary! Janabai said that this sandwich is so popular that it is sold in 40 delis throughout the city.

Next we tucked into a Big Matt "Cheese" Burger, which, without hyperbole, is much the best vegan burger that we've ever tasted, raw or cooked! The patty consisted of a raw mini nut loaf; the cheese was a sunflower seed cheese, and the bun was made from raw onion bread. The trimmings included 6 thin slices of raw, organic pickles, 2 thick tomato slices w 3 leaves of lettuce, a tablespoon of ground mustard; a thin slice of yellow onion and 2 thick tomato slices. This raw burger alone could start a RAWvolution.

Another dish that we relished was their Baby Bok Choy Salad, which was dressed with an emulsion of ginger, garlic, lemon juice, coconut aminos, Himalayan sea salt, and stone-pressed olive oil. It is illustrative of the seemingly endless lengths to which Matt and Janabai are willing to go in order to procure the most healthful and delicious ingredients.

Perhaps the Indonesian Kelp Noodles was the dish that we most savored. Kelp noodles aswim in a chili cashew cream sauce with garlic prepared oil, sprinkled with bits and pieces of bok choy, nori, black sesame seeds, and red peppers. Yummy!

For dessert we had their Jungle Peanut Clusters (Amazon harvested peanuts in a caramel sauce made with yacun syrup that is allowed to harden and set.)Truly exquisite! Between dishes, we quaffed a Green Juice as well as a Vanilla Mint Lemonade which immediately lifted our spirits and lofted RAWvolution among the best juice emporia in the city. Every fortnight, or so, RAWvolution offers a three-day living liquid cleanse. Those who sign up for the cleanse subsist for three days on such beverages as blended fruits; mineralized water; coconut shakes; protein shakes; etc.

If for some reason, you can't make it to either RAWvolution in NYC, or Euphoria Loves RAWvolution in Santa Monica, you might consider ordering The Box. as they call it. Every week Matt creates one of his signature raw dinners to be FedExed to customers who don't wish to stir from their home, or office. This week's box contains raw vegan dishes of Matt's devising such as, Red Russian Borscht; Hearty Lentil Chili; Cauliflower Couscous; Mock Chicken Salad; Cucumber Dill Salad; Greek Pizza; Spinach "Cheese" Quiche; Tostada with Salsa Fresca; Pecan Crumble; and Chocolate Coconut Haystacks. To be sure, it's not inexpensive to have The

Box FedExed to you, but when you stop to consider that The Box costs less than a single entrée at one of New York's high end restaurants like Per Se, or Jean Georges, or DB Bistro Moderne, you'll find it well worth the investment.

The RAWvolution logo is a stylized version of a painting by the famous 19th century *Naturmensch* artist, Fidus. It shows the Edenic couple disporting themselves in paradise. The implication is that eating a vegan raw food diet could transport one to Paradise. Certainly, eating at RAWvolution, we felt we had been given a foretaste of paradise!

'sNICE III [v] $

	150 Sullivan Street
Self service	bet. Prince/ Houston
Sandwiches, salads, baked goods	212-253-5405
All cards	M-F 7:30am-10pm
Beer & wine	Sa-Su 8am-10pm

See description under Greenwich Village

STOGO[ve]$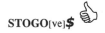

	159 Second Avenue
Counter service	entrance on 10th Street
Gourmet organic vegan ice-cream	(212) 677-2301
Visa & Mastercard	Su-Th 12pm-11pm
No alcohol	Fr-Sa 12pm-12am
www.stogonyc.com	

The third vegan ice-cream store in the US --[The first was Wheeler's Frozen Desserts in Boston,]-- opened on December 5th, 2008. With an eye on a more health conscious alternative to traditional ice cream, Stogo has developed ice cream made from four different bases: Coconut cream, hemp, sorbet and soy. They even make all of their flavors right in their store!

There are baked goods like gluten-free vanilla cupcakes and chocolate chip cookies from Babycakes, and more than 44 flavors of vegan ice cream with more to come! We were immediately struck by how vivid and distinctive those flavors are. The coffee was strong enough to give us a caffeine buzz. The pomegranate tastes as if it had been freshly picked from the trees, as does the mango in the mango sorbet. We are recovering chocoholics, but despite our chocolate-jaded palates, we could actually discern sharp nuances of flavor between the Mexican Spiced Chocolate, the Chocolate Hazelnut, and the Coconut Chocolate. The ingredients are dairy free, gluten-free, and organic. They're also free of artificial flavors and preservatives. As befits such a conscientious vegan establishment, absolutely no animal ingredients are used, and agave nectar is used in lieu of honey and refined sugars. All of their cups and utensils are also biodegradable and compostable. As might be expected, everything is re-cycled including the baked goods from Babycakes. Leftover oatmeal raisin or chocolate chip cookies, for instance, are grist for the ice-cream mill. They're ground into two of Stogo's most fetching flavors—Oatmeal Raisin and Chocolate Chip.

SUSTAINABLE NYC [v] $

Counter service
International
No credit cards
No alcohol
Sustainable-nyc.com

139 Avenue A
at Ninth Street
212-254-5400
M-F 8am-8pm
Sa, Su 9am-8pm

Now customers who wish to lessen their carbon footprint by buying Sustainable New York City's green products--such as biodegradable beauty products; solar backpacks; and chargers for i-pods and blackberries; bio-degradable home cleaning products; recycled stationery, etc.—now, they can shrink their carbon footprint even further by eating at SNYC's in-store café--the vegetarian edition of Ciao for Now.

Ciao for Now, (pun intended) is a family-run restaurant that was started by Amy and Kevin Miceli in 2001. The main location is at 523 East 12th Street between Avenues A and B. Don't look for a review of Ciao For Now in *The Vegan Guide to New York City,* however; because--at its main location and at its other satellite location at 107 W. 10th Street—ruefully, it's not vegetarian.

However, genuflecting to the green ethos of SNYC, Ciao for Now has custom designed a vegetarian menu for its owner, Dominique. We recently chowed at CFN in SNYC starting with the Asian Chop: (Marinated tofu, tarmari almonds, edamame, sprouts, and carrots in a sesame dressing). This is *una bella insalata!* We followed this with a Hummus Sandwich (served on 9-grain bread and filled with carrots, red pepper, sprouts and lettuce). Bravo!

For dessert, we had a tranche of chocolate vegan cake and a Double Chocolate Vegan Espresso Cookie. To wash down the cake and cookie, we sipped a vegan cappuccino (made with fair-trade Ink coffee) that was so savory and smooth that we had doubles on it. In a word, the vegetarian edition of Ciao for Now is a perfect fit for Sustainable NYC.

WHOLE EARTH BAKERY & KITCHEN [ve]]$

Buffet (take-out only)
Organic vegan bakery (some gluten free)
No cards
No alcohol

130 St. Marks Place
bet. First Ave/Avenue A
212-677-7597
Su-Th 9am-12am
F-Sa 9am-1am

Hole-in-the-wall offering organic baked goods and small buffet, wholly vegan. The owner, Peter, is noted for donating his pastries to animal rights events in the city. He assures us that no honey or refined sugar is ever used. Cheeseless pizza, tofu vegetable turnovers, lasagna, eggplant Parmesan; cabbage knishes, soups and puddings along with whole grain baked goodies of the 100% whole wheat, rather dry variety. Almost 50% of his baked goods are gluten-free. Recently, at the Veggie Pride Parade, Peter manned a booth in which he was selling his mixed vegetable Pizzas. There were lines around the block! It's one of the few places left where one may eat to repletion for under ten dollars. For take out mainly—seats four.

SOHO

(Canal Street to Houston Street)

BABYCAKES [ve] $ 👍

Counter service
Vegan baked goods
All cards
No alcohol
www.babycakesnyc.com

248 Broome Street
bet. Orchard/ Ludlow Streets
212-677-5047
Tu-Th 10am-10pm
F 10am-10pm
Su-M 10am-8pm

Although the art-deco, retro interior evokes a roadside diner from the 1920's, unless you're a dessertatarian--as we are--then it's not really possible to have a meal here; however, if you have an overdeveloped sweet tooth--as we do--then you could have a chocolate chip cookie as an appetizer, a carrot cupcake as a main course with some extra frosting on the side [It's $1.50 for a side order of frosting.]--and a slice of pound cake for dessert. You could wash it down with a cup of shade-grown, fair-trade Gorilla coffee, as we did.

Here's a rich irony--the owner, Erin McKenna, is not a vegetarian, but she is scrupulous about not using eggs, or dairy. Instead of honey, she uses stevia and agave nectar --whereas, the techno-pop star Moby, who is a militant vegan, serves eggs, honey and dairy products at his restaurant, Teany, which is only a few blocks away.

Let's face it, there are a lot of excellent vegan and vegetarian restaurants in New York that have execrable desserts--Pukk, Madras Cafe, Vegetarian Dim Sum House, to list but a few. So, have your dinner at Madras Cafe; then saunter over to Babycakes for some sweet, sweet babycakes for dessert. Our current favorites (as of 2010) are the Cinnamon Toastie, plus their new doughnuts—glazed, chocolate, sprinkles and coconut.

LITTLE LAD'S BASKET [v] $ 👍

Self service, buffet
International
No cards
No alcohol

41 Delancey Street
at Essex Street
212-227-5744
Daily 9am-9pm

Like Dr. John "Cornflakes" Kellogg, Larry, the owner of Little Lad's is a 7th-Day Adventist, who is on a mission to convert the world to vegetarianism one-meal at a time. However, he makes it plain that he is not funded by the Adventist Church. They encourage him but they don't provide him with any financial backing.[Did we detect a trace of acrimony in his admission?]

Larry has used the same formula in creating the Little Lad's chain--{He envisages it as a globe-girdling chain of vegetarian restaurant franchises.)--that he used in his previous restaurant venture--Country Life, which was a veg.restaurant chain that once girdled the US and Europe in the early 1990's. Successful, though it was, it failed from exuberant over-expansion. It was wildly popular during its heyday in New York and Boston. People still remember it wistfully.

We had a vegan mock Shepherd's Pie, a vegan French Onion Soup, and a Cheeseless Cheese Cake. All delicious and all for only $4.99.Larry, who mans the register, took our money. Judging from the high quality and low price of the food here, Little Lad's will be around at least until the Second Advent.

• At the end of 2011, Little Lad's moved from the Financial District to the Lower East Side.

ORGANIC AVENUE-3 [ve] $$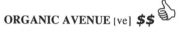

Self service	156 Sullivan Street
Organic raw food bar/boutique	bet. West Houston / Prince Street

ORGANIC AVENUE [ve] $$

Full service	116 Suffolk Street
Organic raw food boutiaue	bet. Delancey/ Rivington Streets
All major cards	212-358-0500
No alcohol	M-F 8am-8pm
www.organicavenue.com	Sa,Su 8am-10pm

Time was when Organic Avenue sold hemp clothing, organic lifestyle products, books, organic vegan snacks, as well as organic fruits and vegetables. They still do, but the raw organic fruits and vegetables have given way to organic raw fruit and vegetable juices and smoothies along with chef-crafted raw food dishes.

It was when founder-owner, Denise Mari met her husband Doug, an astute vegan businessman, that they started to focus intently on selling cold pressed organic raw juices, smoothies, and raw organic vegan prepared foods. The juices, smoothies, and foods were dispensed in containers and sold in refrigerator cases. In late 2010, they hired gourmet raw food chef, Peter Cerevon-- who had trained under raw food chef Chad Sarno, of Vital Creations—to imbue OA's organic vegan raw food with his authority and culinary flair.

We quaffed a Blueberry Smoothie and followed it with a Portobello Sandwich. For dessert, we ate their Coco-Lime Pie. All were surpassingly yummy. Unusually, after such a heavy meal, we felt strangely lifted and energized.

While I browsed the raw food books, my companion tried on a pastel top, which was on sale for half price. At Organic Avenue, there is a juxtaposition of food, books, and clothing that gratified all our appetites save one. All in all, luncheon at OA was a thoroughly engaging way to wile away an afternoon.

PUNJAB [v] $
Counter service
Indian fast food
No cards
No alcohol

114 East First Street
at Avenue A
212-533-9048
daily 24 hours

This unprepossessing samosa shack is hard to find, but worth a look-in. It's located in the basement of a building on East First Street with an awning that is misleadingly labeled as a deli-grocery. Down the stairs, one spies Indian cabdrivers munching on samosas, rotis and other vegetarian delights. We mimicked them and ordered a Tikki (potato pancake) slathered with chickpeas and told the counterman that we wanted it without milk, cheese or ghee. Like everyone else in this bustling, cramped place--we ate it standing up. It went down very well.

In the refrigerated display case, there are other pre-cooked curry dishes that just need to be heated in the microwave to be revived. We tried the Curried Bitter Melon, and found it astringent but tasty. The fact that cabbies eat here is a good sign. Typically, cabbies seek out the most flavorful and frugal vegetarian food. So their presence is almost a guarantee of a satisfying meal, however hurried.

TEANY [v] $

Full service
International
All cards)
Beer & wine

90 Rivington Street
bet. Orchard/ Ludlow
212-475-9190
W, Th, Su 10am-10pm
F, Sa 10am-2am

Teany is a restaurant-cum-teahouse that was founded by the rock star Moby. Its name, Teany, stands for Tea New York, but it is also a pun, referring wryly to its diminutive size. It's teeny as well as teany.

The portions, however, are ample. For instance the faux turkey club sandwich, which we adored, is big enough to feed two people; and the salads, the crostini, and the granola dishes are as generous as they are delicious. Along with the Club Sandwich, we recommend the Crostini. Thin toast ovals are served with four vegan spreads--Olive, White Bean, Artichoke and Herbed Soy Cheese. It's big of Teany that after you've dipped all your toast ovals in the pots of vegan spreads, Teany will freely replenish them.

Teany desserts are tremendous! We particularly liked the Tofu Chocolate Cheese Cake, and the Peanut Butter Chocolate cake, which are supplied to Teany by the Vegan Treats bakery. The eponymous tea menu is as extensive as any four star restaurant's wine list. Last time we were there, we savored the black tea called Golden Monkey,. but there are uncaffeinated herb teas as well. Sad to report: we found the homemade sodas to be flavorless and insipid.

Although Moby is co-owner of the restaurant with his ex-girlfriend Kelly Tisdale, he likens himself to a Victorian father who sees the baby only now and then. He writes the checks but Kelly does the day-to-day running of the shop. In providing such delicious fare in such a tastefully designed space, however teeny--Moby has done the community a whale of a service. Incidentally, Moby, (nee Richard Melvile Hall), is nicknamed after the whale in his distant ancestor, Herman Melvile's novel Moby Dick. He is a committed vegan; one could only wish that he had extended his veganism to the entire menu. Vegan dishes are marked with an asterisk.

TIEN GARDEN [ve] $$ 👍

Full service
Chinese Homestyle
All cards
No alcohol

170 Allen Street
at E. Houston/ 1st Avenue
212-388-1364
M-Sa 12pm-10pm

Not so long ago, Tiengarden was a lonely outpost of veganism on the lower East Side. Now it may be seen as something of a neighborhood trendsetter. Within the past two years it has become surrounded by eco-conscious stores like Earth Matters and Bluestockings; tony vegan boutiques like MooShoes, and Organic Avenue; and fashionable vegetarian restaurants like Teany.

Based on the ancient theory of five elements--metal, water, earth, and fire--the food at Tiengarden is prepared in such a way as to maximize its chi, or life force. On the other hand, foods that are considered to be sapping of one's chi are scrupulously avoided. So in addition to being vegan, (because animal products are considered to be deleterious to one's chi); the dishes contain no garlic, or onions, which are also held to be harmful to one's chi. Nonetheless, the food is quite delectable without these flavor intensifiers.

We are partial to their Pan-Fried Bean Curd Sandwich, their Mixed Gluten Salad (Spicy braised wheat gluten is served on a bed of lettuce with tomato, celery and carrot sticks and served with a vegan barbecue sauce or vegan mayo.); their Special Nuggets (soy nuggets, red bell peppers, broccoli, cauliflower, zucchini, cashews in a light curry peanut sauce). We also ate with gusto their Basil Beancurd (crisp, layered beancurd with broccoli, tomato and mushrooms in basil sauce).

Unlike most Chinese restaurants, desserts here are totally vegan, substantial, and delicious.,Our current favorite is the Banana Surprise. Fresh bananas surround generous glops of soy ice-cream.) And, like the rest of the food, even their home-made fresh pies and cakes are chi-enhancing.

WILD GINGER [v] $$ 👍

Full service
Pan-Asian
All cards
Beer, wine & sake
www. wildgingervegan.com

380 Broome Street
bet. Mott/ Mulberry Streets
212-966-1883/ 2669
daily 12pm-11pm

Three friends--Richard, (the architect and co-manager), Winnie (the accountant and manager), and her husband, Tim (the chef)--have pooled their assets, as it were, to create one of the most

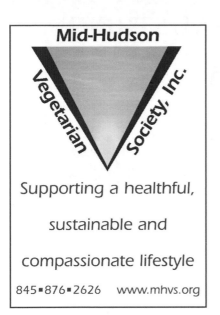
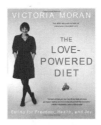
popular and successful vegetarian restaurants in town. Richard is responsible for the elegant yet cozy interior; Winnie, for the crisply efficient running of the place; and Tim for the tasty dishes. "Pan Asian" is how they describe their cuisine--Thai, Chinese, Malaysian and Indian--and for once the menu truly deserves this overused and often inaccurate appellation.

We practically shouted our adulation of the Scallion Pancakes with the Home-Made Mango Salsa, which tasted less like crepes than small pizzas topped with a piquant mango sauce. We adored the Samosa in Curry Sauce. Their newest appetizer, Tempeh in Satay Sauce is supernal. For the main course, our taste buds thrilled to the exotic flavor notes in Malaysian Curry Stew (Mild, Slow-Cooked Coconut Curry with Soy Protein, Broccoli, Carrots, Potatoes and Pumpkin). and Mango Soy Protein (Thin-Slice Medallions Sautéed in a Mellow Plum Sauce with Mango, Zucchini, Sweet-Sage Turnips, Peppers, and Onions).

Beverages--we tossed off the homemade Wild Ginger Beer, and Virgin Mojitoes with gusto. They were--at least to our teetotal, non-alcoholic sensibilities-- bewitching. For drinkers of more adult beverages, there is an array of beers, wine and sakes that are guaranteed to "bewitch, bother and bewilder." Vegans, however, should beware the Lassis (an Indian drink made with fruit juice and yogurt). Order soy-milk Lassis instead!

Chef Tim accrued his repertoire of Pan-Asian vegan dishes by working in a string of different veg. restaurants--such as Zen Palate, Tien Garden and assorted others--as a sous-chef. But by now, Tim has clearly outstripped his masters; so while one may recognize many of the menu dishes from having dined elsewhere, seldom have they been prepared to such palate-pleasing perfection.

BELOW CANAL STREET
(Includes Chinatown, Tribeca, Financial District)

BUDDHA BODAI VEGETARIAN RESTAURANT [v] **$$**

Full service	5 Mott Street
Chinese (kosher)	at Bowery
All cards	212-566-8388
No alcohol.	daily 10:30am-10:30pm

See description under Queens

HOUSE OF VEGETARIAN [v] **$** 👍

Full service	68 Mott Street
Chinese Homestyle	bet. Canal/Bayard Streets
No cards	212-226-6572
11pm	daily 11am
Beer & wine	

This is one Chinatown restaurant where there aren't any fresh kills hanging in the window. "All We Are Served Vegetarian Dishes" reads the reassuring note on the extensive menu of more than 200 dishes, from Vegetarian Roast Duck (too much of a poultry flavor for our taste) to Braised Chicken with Lily Flowers (made from wheat gluten) or everybody's favorite, Iron Steak, made from yams and quite tasty. Our own personal favorite were mock Chicken with Mango and Black Mushrooms With Soysticks. Served in a narrow dining room with plastic tablecloths and no ambiance, but the food's good and there's plenty of it.

VEGETARIAN DIM SUM HOUSE [ve] **$$** 👍

Full service	24 Pell Street
Chinese	at Mott Street
No cards	212-577-7176
No alcohol	daily 11am-11pm

Vegetarian Dim Sum House serves most of the same dishes that its sister restaurant, House of Vegetarian, serves except that it offers them amid posher surroundings with a wider range of dim sum dishes. "Dim Sum" (literally "cooked snacks") are the snack-like dishes that are popular in Hong Kong, Taiwan and other parts of South China. The Cantonese like to put together several dim sum dishes for breakfast, lunch and tea; they even have a few dim sum dishes as appetizers before dinner. Because they may eat dim sum three or four times a day, these snacks have to be skillfully prepared to avoid boring the jaded palate. The dim sum that we had at the Dim Sum House were certainly unboring. We particularly liked the Spinach Dumpling, the Lotus Root Cake, and the Sticky Rice wrapped in Lotus Leaf. From the main course menu, we liked the mock roast duck and the mock chicken dishes made from tofu skin. Portions are generous and service is attentive.

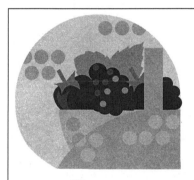

Congratulations:

The Vegan Guide to New York City

On Your 18th Anniversary!
Keep Up the Excellent Work!

...Compliments of a Friend

BROOKLYN

BLISS [v] $$

Full service
Natural
No cards
No alcohol

191 Bedford Avenue
bet. N6th / N7th Streets
718-599-2547
daily 8am-11pm

"Bliss was it in that dawn to be alive and eating brunch at Bliss, but to be vegetarian was very heaven!" is what Wordsworth might have written had he been a vegetarian and had he had the good fortune to dine at Bliss--one of New York's better vegetarian restaurants. He would surely have waxed poetic over the vegan BLT.'s that are made with Fakin' Bacon, the Veggie Burgers and the Seitan "Steak" Sandwiches. The salads are a tone poem and the desserts an ode to Bliss. With prices so much lower in Williamsburg than for comparable fare in Manhattan, it's worth hopping the L train and traveling East just one stop from Manhattan for so much more bliss for the buck.
    • Recent visits, in late 2011, yielded less bliss for the buck, but it's still worth a subway jaunt.

BODY AND SOUL[ve] $

Food stand
International, organic
No cards
No alcohol

Farmers' Market
at Grand Army Plaza
212-982-5870
Sa 8am-4pm
Sa 8am-4pm

One of the best ways to keep body and soul together in the city is to have a light vegan meal at the vegan food stand in the Grand Army Plaza Farmers' market., which is called aptly enough Body and Soul. Started by the owners of Counter restaurant back in 1994, it draws throngs of hungry folk for breakfast, lunch, early light suppers, and snacks. And it's easy to see why. The out-size wraps and turnovers are scrumptious. Try the Saffron Potato wrap which teases the palate with plantain chunks hidden inside. Or try the Spinach Portabello Turnover, which is filled with tofu ricotta, and tastes a bit like a Spinach Lasagna. You might want to complement this with a dairy-free Blueberry Muffin, Or a Sweet Potato Muffin. Don't leave the stand without biting into a melt-in-your-mouth Chocolate Brownie, or a Wheat-Free Almond Cookie. Then repair to one of the benches in Prospect Park and have an *al fresco* meal.

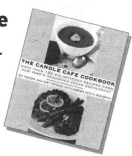

BONESHAKERS [v] $ 👍

Conterl service
Sandwich & salad cafe
Cash only
Beer, wine & sake
www.brooklynboneshakers.com

134 Kingsland Avenue
at Beadel [Williamsbug]
718-963-0656
M-F 8an-10on
Sa-Su 9an-9on

Boneshakers! An odd name for a vegetarian restaurant! It sounds like a Halloween *danse macabre*. In fact, Boneshakers, the restaurant was started by two cycling enthusiasts. Megan Blackburn and Brad Baker. They told us that "boneshakers" was the name given to the first bicycle. Its pedals--instead of being attached to a drive train--were attached directly to the front wheel, making it wobbly and unstable, making it a real boneshaker!! Boneshaker is also something of a *double entendre* in that it refers to the strong coffee that they serve here in a variety of blends. It is supplied by the Gimme Coffee Co., a neighborhood purveyor. In fact, the motto of Boneshakers, emblazoned on a sign that hangs in the window is "Death Before Decaf." Their iced coffee--which in our opinion is their best brew-- is made from grounds that are soaked for twelve hours. The resultant concentrate it then poured into a glass with ice and soymilk and served. It too causes the bones to rattle, roll and shake!

Cycling posters and pictures of cycling champions like Eddy Merckx, and the great Molteni adorn the walls. Most of the sandwiches and salads are named after top cyclists like the legendary Merckx, "The Hill Bomber" which refers to Magnus, the stoutest cyclist on the current professional tour who weighs in at 200 plus pounds. They call him Magnus for short.

We opted for the Rebel Cruiser which contained BBQ Seitan with coleslaw and served on a Kaiser bun. We also munched the Koichi, named for the Japanese track racing champion, who won ten successive world championships (avocado, sprouts, chipotle vegan mayo, served on a Kaiser roll).

For dessert, we downed an incredibly delicious vegan Danish pastry, which was supplied by their exqusited vegan patisserie, located just blocks away, called Champs. As purveyors of delicious veg. food, Brad and Megan rank among the champs.

CHAMPS [ve]] $ 👍

Conterl service
Sandwich & salad cafe
Cash only
No alcohol
www.champsbakeryscom

176 Ainsle Street
at Leonard Street [Williamsbug]
718-599-2743
M-Sa 12pm-10pm
Su 12pm-6pm

The aptly named "Champs" is the undisputed champion among the vegan bakeries in NYC. For complex pastries such as croissants, cinnamon swirls, and Danish pastries, they are simply unrivaled. While brunching there, we met one of the Champ bakers, a lady named Evan, who is a real craftsman of baked comestibles. At her suggestion, we tried the three-berry-filled Danish. We haven't had Danish since childhood, but this was the best Danish we've ever tasted, ever!

Next, we had chocolate cinnamon swirls. We also munched a chocolate chip cookie whose chips are impeccably vegan (from Tropical Source). As any self-respecting vegan toll house cookie should be, they were chewy and gooey and crunchy-but Champs' are a cut above the rest.. We chased all those sweet comestibles with Gimme Fair Trade Iced Coffee (which they soak rather than brew). We left the bakery feeling as if we were vegan fly-weight champs of the world.

DAO PALATE VEGAN [v] $$

Full service
Pan Asian
All cards
Beer, wine & sake
www. Daopalatevegan.com

201 5th Avenue
bet. Sackett/ Union Streets
718-622-2088
daily 12pm-10:45pm

DAO PALATE [v] $$

Full service
Pan Asian
All cards
Beer, wine & sake
www. Daopalate.com

329 Flatbush Avenue
at Seventh Avenue
718-638-1995/1998
N-Th 12pm -11:pm
F-Su 12pm-11:30pm
Su 12pm-10:30pm

If you have eaten at any of the wonderful Wild Ginger restaurants in the city [There are three altogether.]--you will have a sense of déjà vu when you dine at Dao Palate. The menu is almost identical to that of Wild Ginger. This duplication has come about because the owner of Tao Palate, Yuan-Yao Dong, is a distant relative of the co-owner of two other Wild Gingers. The story is a family saga that is far too convoluted to be deconstructed here. Suffice it to say that the cuisine, which Yuan-Yao describes as "Pan-Asian," [Malaysian, Indian, Korean, Japanese and Chinese], is several cuts above the rest.

On entering, we were struck by the three statues of the Buddha that smile beneficently on the non-violent feeding. The room is tastefully decorated with hammered brass sculptures on the exposed brick walls.

We started with crispy vegetable tofu skin wraps with tangy sauce, that were addictively tasty. Then we had the Mango Soy Protein with Vegetables in Plum Sauce, which was sumptuously exotic to the taste. This was accompanied by Pineapple Fried Rice, which we particularly prized because the pineapple, broccoli, and avocado chunks were flash-cooked so that they retained their true flavors. For dessert, we had their delectable Three-Berry Cheese Cake, in which the flavor of each berry seemed to be individuated.

We closed the meal with a mug of fair trade coffee, lightened with soy-milk, and sweetened with agave nectar. As we sipped this warm beverage, it struck us forcibly that the restaurant was aptly named: Tao (the ideal path) for the Palate.

•On a recent visit we found that the quality and service had fallen off. The dishes were rushed out, perfunctorily prepared; and the waitress removed our plates before we were done. They were more interested in turning over the table than providing good service. The check was also foisted on us before we had finished our desserts.

FOODSWINGS [ve] $

Counter service	295 Grand Street
Fast food	bet. Roebling/ Havemeyer
All cards	718-388-1919
No alcohol	Su-Th 11:30am-12am
	F, Sa 11:30am-2am

Foodswings underwent a change of ownership--and a change of appearance--in early 2009.The former owner, Freedom Tripodi had put his unique eatery on the auction block. Happily, it was purchased by dedicated vegans with business acumen—Jeff and Hope--who are also owners of New York's (and possibly the world's) only vegan saloon--Lucky 13 (in Park Slope). Co-owner, Jeff Blanchard, is also a bassist, vocalist and founding member of the rock group, Eyes of the Sun.

Recently we swung by to see how the new Foodswings stacked up against the old. We're delighted to report that the animal rights spirits that pervaded the old Foodswings are still palpable. The walls are festooned with PETA posters; and brochures from nearby animal sanctuaries still abound.

Not incidentally, they still serve the best French fries in the cosmos! [Studies have shown that people go to the Golden Arches and other burger joints mainly for the French fries.] Their mock Chicken Cutlet sandwich on a Kaiser bun is still as tasty as it ever was. We also noted some improvements: They now make their own seitan from scratch; so that the flavor of their Homemade Chili Con Seitan is greatly enhanced by it. They make their Grilled Cheese Sandwich; their Mock Ham and Cheese Sandwich--along with many of their other sandwiches that contain mock cheese--with vegan Daiya Cheese. Made from cassava (tapioca), it's gooier and cheesier than any other ersatz cheese we've tasted.

Still the best-selling item on the menu, their Gyro-- (Seasoned mock beef with lettuce, tomato, red onion with vegan Tzatziki sauce.)—rules! Although we prefer their Sausage & Pepper Hero (Homemade vegan Italian sausage with peppers and onions on Italian bread.)

What's fast food without a soy-milkshake chaser? We chased ours with a Pistachio Shake (their Basic Shake with vegan pistachio ice-cream). They've increased the seating capacity of the room and have added a bathroom, the lack of which was one of the few drawbacks of the old Foodswings. Yes, dear reader, the new Foodswings is truly a swinging place to eat!

FOUR SEASONS RESTAURANT [ve} $

	2281 Church Avenue
Counter service	at Bedford Avenue
Caribbean vegetarian	718-693-7996
$4.00-10.00 [no cards}	M-Th 9am-10pm
No alcohol	Fr-Sa 9am-12; Su 11am-7pm

This is not to be confused with the higher rent, higher cholesterol restaurant of the same name in

Manhattan. This is the healthier vegetarian version. It's Fresh Assorted Curries, Vegetarian Lo Mein, Vegan Baked Goods and Fresh-Squeezed Juices will delight your palate and are guaranteed to ward off a thrombosis.

IMHOTEPS [ve] $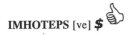

Self service
West Indian vegetarian, organic
No cards
No alcohol

734 Nostrand Ave.
bet. Park Place & Prospect
718-493-2395
daily- 8:30am-12am

Imhoteps is the name of an Egyptian minister during the reign of the pharaoh Zoser, who ruled Egypt about 2650 BCE. Imhotep's wisdom was so vast that he has been deified as the creator of medicine and the epitome of sagacity. The owners of this Brooklyn eatery--Tonde and Maketa-- named both their first son and their restaurant after this legendary Egyptian sage. Had Imhoteps been a chef then he could not have crafted a tastier or a healthier cuisine than the food that is on offer at Imhoteps. The chef Victor Telesford was the founding chef at Veggie Castle, and his skill at the stove did a lot to make Veggie Castle the roaring success that it is today. The food is so seductive that many customers eat three meals a day here. Among the dishes that are especially recommended are Soy Salmon and Vegie Roast Duck, but everything on the menu is mouth-watering. The beverages, which include protein shakes, sorrel, wheat grass and sea-moss juices are healthful and bracing. We had a glass of Sorrel with our Soy Salmon and Veggie Roast Duck and topped off our meal with a Carrot Sea Moss vegan ice cream that was laced with gingko--the memory enhancing herb--that made the whole culinary experience even more unforgettable.

PERELANDRA [v] $

Counter service
Internatinal
All Cards
No alcohol
www. perelandra natural.com

175 Remsen Street
bet. Court/ Clinton
718-855-6068
M-F 8:30-8:30
Sa 9:30-8:30:
Su 11-7

On their way to work, Brooklyn's pinstripe brigade pauses here just long enough to scarf down the Breakfast Sandwich, which is Perelandra's answer to the ghastly EggMaguffin (sic.). The Perelandra version consists of baked tofu, tempeh bacon, avocado, dill, and caramelized onion served on a Freshly Baked Spelt Muffin. Yummmy! Organic oatmeal with a different fresh fruit is served daily.

The pinstriped set returns for lunch, and it is not uncommon to see a long line of men and women in business suits standing politely in a line that insinuates itself through the store (Brooklyn's largest health food store). With courts and investment houses hard by, we are in

Brooklyn's legal and business district. Eaten up with curiosity, we eavesdropped on the line-waters'c onversations: Sure enough, torts as well as tortes were being hotly discussed.

Every day Perelandra's menu changes, but the categories remain the same. For instance, every day they offer a Soup; a Sauce and Grain, A Casserole a Sandwich: a Wrap; an Entree and a Dessert.

For lunch we slurped their fresh Miso Soup; then savored the Japanese Wasabi Potato Salad and a Barbecue Un-Chicken Sandwich. We also sampled their Baked Vegetable Risotto. For the grand finale, we downed their inimitable Tofu Vegan Cheesecake. For the post prandial beverage, we sipped their Avocado Smoothie. Which contains Coconut Juice, Avocado, Agave Nectar, and Fresh Lime Juice. We specifically requested that they make it with Agave nectar as they ordinarily make it with honey. After the ethical sweetener were added, we tossed it off with gusto! Replete with delilcous vegan food and drink, we wobbled through the store's portal into a sun-splashed Brroklyn summer afteroon.

RAW STAR [v] $$ 👍

Counter service	687 Washington Avenue
Raw West Indian Cuisine	bet. St. Marks/ Prospect
No Cards	718-975-0304
No alcohol	Tu-Sa 11am-11pm
wwwrawstarcafe.com	Su 9am-11pm

The newest star in the firmament of rawfood restaurants is Mawule Job Simon's Raw Star. The décor is reminiscent of Mawule's ill-starred venture, Green Paradise, which opened iin 2003, but went kaput in 2004 because it was too far ahead of its time. From Green Paradise, Mawule has salvaged the counter made from palm wood and thatched palm fronds, which he built by himself (proving that he is as handy with a hammer and saw as he is with a spatula). The chartreuse walls are festooned with works of art, the most striking of which s a painting depicting scantily clad rawfoodists frolicking in an African Eden. The background music consists of reggae versions of popular tunes--to the strains of which we ate our sumptuous meal.

A native of Trinidad, Mawule, earned his stripes as a raw chef by training at Brooklyn's now defunct SunFire juice Club with the legendary Aris La Tham, America's first vegan rawfood gourmet chef.

Aris has since decamped to Jamaica where he runs a Sunfired Spa in Ochos Rios. The best way to taste Aris' food without traveling to Ocho Rios is to eat at Raw Star. Mawule pays homage to his mentor by including a few of Aris's signature dishes on the menu. Such s Tree Fruit, Curried Plantain, Tain. Whis Salad and the ineffable Banana Cream Pie.

But Mawule is an innovative rawfood chef in is own right. He adds a Trinidadian fillip to the dishes that delight and deceive the palate.

Many of his dishes are *trompe l'oeil* for the tongue. For instance, his raw Tabouleh is actually made with cauliflower florets that are prepared to look like grains of cracked wheat. Similarly, he makes a raw tempeh dish which really isn't tempeh, but is made from a variety of unfired vegetables. The artfully prepared dishes tease and titillate the palate. The dessert, which pays tribute to the master, Aris La Tham, that we favored is his raw Banana Cream Pie. Its flavor notes along with those of almost every other dish on the menu at Raw Star are positively celestial.

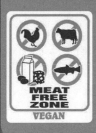
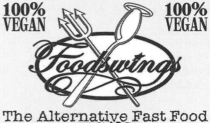
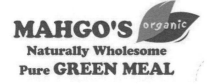

ROCKIN' RAW [v] *$$*

Full service   178 N. Eighth St.
Peruvian-New Orleanian raw food   bet. Bedford / Driggs Avenues
All major cards   718-599-9333
Full bar   T-Sa 3pm-10pm
www.rockinraw.com   Su 1pm-9pm

Luis Salgado of Lima, Peru and Tere Fox of New Orleans, Louisiana met at a rock concert, and shortly thereafter, they enrolled as students at the Institute of Integrative Nutrtition, of which they are alumni. Soon after graduating, they decided to merge their talents and their knowledge of their native cuisines to open a restaurant where they and their executive chef, Vanessa Cabrera, have created some of the most innovative vegan rawfoods dishes in the city.

Tere ushered us into the garden, which is lushly landscaped, and so serene that birds flock to it as though it were a sanctuary. [Perhaps they sensed that none of their winged cousins were on the menu.]

We commenced with the Mushroom Cebiche. (Crimini mushrooms; white mushrooms; onions; and a roma tomato are marinated in a spicy citrus sauce.) It was a piquant foretaste of delicious dishes to come.

Next we tucked into a Louisiana Gumbo which contains one of our favorite vegetables (actually a fruit)--okra. Topped with a sprinkling of cauliflower florets (an ersatz raw rice), a smoky-tasting mock sausage is set a-swim in a spicy, gooey, gumbo base that was tangy and flavorful.

Between bites, we slaked our thirst with a Cucumber Mojito, and a Watermelon Cooler which were utterly refreshing--followed by a Chocolate and a Strawberry Smoothie (made with home-made almond milk) which were most exhilarating.

We then fell upon the Raw Boy Sandwich with Cajun Mayo. This is a raw vegan version of the classic New Orleans "Po Boy." Faux raw tuna is served between two slices of home-made Essene bread, and slathered with a cajun mayo. It is served with a side dish of Creole Cole Slaw, and Flax Crackers. We found it to be much the best item on the menu and instantly nominated it as one of the two best sandwiches of the year (along with Peacefood Café's Horn Mushroom Panini).

The dessert we selected was Lucuma Ice-Cream topped with Fudge Sauce, and a Lucuma vegan cheesecake. Lucuma is a tropical fruit with a delicate flavor that is native to Peru. Clearly the dishes at Rockin' Raw are correlative of the owners, Louis and Terre, in that they commingle Peruvian and Lousianian accemts. Furthermore, if Rockin' Raw proves to be the success that it promises to be, Terre and Luis plan to open branches of Rockin' Raw in both Lima and New Orleans. Let's help them become the Rockin' success that they deserve to be.

Indicates we especially recommend this restaurant for the quality of the food

'sNICE II [v] $

315 5th Avenue
at 3rd Street
718-788-2121
daily 7:30am-10pm

Self service
Sandwiches, salads, baked goods
All cards
Beer & wine

See description under Greenwich Village

STRICTLY VEGETARIAN [ve] $

2268 Church Avenue
bet.Bedford/Flatbush Avenues
718-284-2543
daily noon-11:30pm

Counter service
Carribean vegetarian
$4.00-8.00 (no cards)
No alcohol

Just down the street from the late Veggie Castle with which it can stand comparison, this place serves such delicious Caribbean vegetarian dishes as Chick Pea Stew, Vegetable Chow Mein and Tofu Stew. The menu changes daily.

SUN IN BLOOM [ve] $$

460 Bergen Street
bet. Flatbush/ Fifth Avenues
718-622-4303
dairly 8am-8pm
Brunch Sa-Su

Full service
Organic vegan gourmet
All cards
www. suninbloom.com

Amy Follette used to run the Bikram Yoga School in Park Slope for 5 years. Where she also counseled her yoga students (and a few outside clients) on adopting a plant based diet, which is a prerequisite of classic yoga training. Though fulfilled in her work, she always had an urge to open a vegan restaurant. Then last January, Organic Heights went out of business, and she had an option to open a restaurant on the vacant site. So she sprang at the chance.

Bikram's loss is our gain, because the food that she prepares at Sun In Bloom may be described only with superlatives.

We started with Irresistible Granola Delight--a kefir with coconut milk base---to which she had added a vegan granola and chopped peaches. Divine!

Then we tucked into her Bloom Burger- a live burger made with sprouted, dehydrated sunflower seeds, and cabbage, layered with fresh tomatoes, crunchy, caramelized onions, and slathered with a live ranch dressing. It was much the best burger, we've ever tasted, raw or cooked.

Next we had her Reuben Special which features "corned" tempeh with a mountain of live sauerkraut, served with a kitchen-fresh Russian dressing with a dash of dulse. Sublime!

While we downed our food, we sipped two terrific smoothies--an Acai Punch, which consisted of acia, raw apple cider vinegar, soymilk, frozen bananas and strawberries that really packed a punch. We also quaffed her Ambrosia Smoothie (young coconut, raw cacao, raw goji berries, raw almond butter, coconut kefir yogurt, banana, and strawberries.) Truly ambrosial!

For dessert we had a live Peach Cheesecake composed of a cashew cheese, and fresh peaches.

Amy is on a mission to get people to eat food that is directly created from photosynthesis--Sun Food ,as it were--rather than being filtered through the bodies of animals. Judging from the high quality of her food, the hygienic freshness of her sun-splashed restaurant, she is poised for success.

• On a recent visit to SIB, a little more than a year after they opened,, we found that they had installed a restroom, and expanded their brunch menu, which is available on weekends from10am-5pm. We sampled one of their brunch specials, which has proved so popular that it is now featured on their regular menu. This was their gluten free pancake stack. Topped with caramelized bananas, seasonal fruit and a splash of maple syrup, it went down very well.

V-SPOT CAFE, THE [ve] *$$*

	156 Fifth Avenue
Full service	bet. Douglass/ Degraw Streets
Latin cuisine	718-622-2275
All cards	T-Th 11am -10:pm
Beer & wine	F-Su 11am-11pm
thevspotcafe.com	Brunch Sa-Su 11am-4pm

Verily an erogenous zone for the vegan palate is Daniel Carabano's new Park Slope vegan eatery called the "V-spot." Here the dishes are. in the uncensored words of a lady friend, who dines there often--"Sooooo gooood!" We certainly wanted to have what she was having; so we ventured over to the V-Spot to see what all the fuss and bother was about. There in an intimate room, with the artwork of local Brooklyn artists adorning exposed brick walls, we savored the V-Spot experience.

Serious vegans, will be impressed by the V-Spot's dedication to ethical standards. The menu proclaims: "All of our dishes are strictly vegetarian. That is, they do not contain any meat chicken, fish, eggs, milk, cheese, honey, casein, gelatin, whey or any other animal or animal derived product. Our mock meat products are meatless and contain soy." Clearly the V in this V-Spot is not for Vendetta, but for Victory!

Dan, the owner, who often doubles as a waiter, took our order. A high-school math-teacher-turned-vegan restaurateur, Dan is a true Pythagorean. [Pythagoras--as you were probably not instructed in your high school geometry classes--founded a society for the study of mathematics in ancient Greece which required that its initiates be strict vegetarians or vegans.]

Most of the dishes on the menu are based on family recipes--such as the appetizer

Empanadas--that Dan inherited from his Colombian paternal grandmother. Even the seemingly prosaic Steak with Rice & Beans (Bandeja Paisa)--is reminiscent of the authentic *comida* to be had in the village cantinas of South America. Its authenticity--albeit veganized,--is why it, and so many of the other dishes with a Latin flair, are so utterly transporting.] Recently, Dan has installed a fresh jjuice bar, and is now offering raw and gluten-free options.

The Latin flair extends to Italian specialties such as Whole-wheat Lasagna, "Chicken" Ptarmigan, Quinoa Pasta Marinara, Pesto Portabella Panini, and the Veggie Tacos that danced fandangos on our tongue. Piquant also were the side orders of Spinach with Garlic and Oil; Plantains; Sweet Potato Fries, and Cury Chickpeas and Kale. To the latest menu, Dan has added two superb new dishes. An appetizer Raw Nori Rolls (A ginger almond pate surrounds a center of spinach and carrots) plus a new entree: Tofu Thai Curry. Desserts are the dependably scrumptious vegan treats from Vegan Treats Bakery as well as a bright array of vegan ice-creams. The V-Spot is successfully retailing its most popular food items at health food stores and delis throughout the five boroughs. These items include their Colombian Empanadas, Curried Quinoa with Kale, Lasagna, Pad Thai, Seitan Burritos, Sesame Quinoa Wrap., and Sesame Tofu. Many of Dan's creations are available through the online grocer, Fresh Direct at www. Freshdirect.com,

VEGETARIAN GINGER   [v] $$

128 Montague Street (2nd Fl)
Full service   Corner Montague/ Henry Streets
Chinese   718-246-1288
All cards   M-Th 11:30am-10:30pm
No alcohol   Fr, Sa 11:30am,-11:00pm
                                 Su: 12:00--10:00pm

It's great to see a new vegan Chinese restaurant on the site of the old Greens [a quondam vegan Chinese restaurant at the same location.], however, one wishes they weren't so derivative--in their title and in the quality of their food. There are already two Wild Gingers in Brooklyn and one Vegetarian Palate. So having one more Chinese vegan restaurant with ginger in the title merely adds to he confusion. Couldn't they have been a bit more inventive and called themselves something else? Jade Pumpkin? Red Persimmon? The Pink Fig? The Golden Peach? The food is flavorful here, and we particularly enjoyed the Smoked Teriyaki Seitan and the Jade Mushrooms, but the dishes, like the name of the restaurant itself, are lacking in originality

VEGETARIAN PALATE   [v] $$

258 Flatbush Avenue
Full service   Bet Prospect Park/ St. Marks
Chinese   718-623-8809
All cards   M-Th 11:30am-11pm
No alcohol   Fr, Sa 11:30am,-11:30pm
                                 Su: 12:00--11:00pm

Vegetarian Palate probably has the most extensive menu of any vegetarian restaurant in the city. Which reminds us of the famous adage that you should never fall in love with someone who has more problems that you, or play cards with someone named "Doc," or eat in a restaurant named "Mom's,"--or in one that has a superabundance of items on the menu. Like most Chinese vegan restaurants Vegetarian Palate abounds in mock meats--as witness their vegetarian seafood dish, Ocean Harvest, which features a collection of vegetarian shrimp, scallops, and squid served with broccoli, snow peas, and baby corn. But the ultimate mock meat tour de force is their Paella Valencia , which is composed of sundry mock seafoods such as shrimp, scallops, crab, mock chicken, mock eel, tofu, shitake mushrooms with mixed vegetables. The service is crisply efficient, the decor, garish. Other diners have complained of excessive starch and oil in the dishes, but one may request of the waiter that these additives be omitted. We had the Soy Chicken with Spinach in Curry Sauce, and the Soy Lemon Chicken and our palates were beguiled by them. For dessert we indulged ourselves in a Banana Split, made with three scoops of non-dairy ice-cream covered with sprinkles and chocolate syrup--all of which soothed our vegetarian palate.

WILD GINGER II [v] *$$*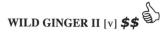

	212 Bedford Avenue
Full service	at North 5th Street
Pan-Asian	718-218-8828

WILD GINGER III [v] *$$*

	112 Smith Street
Full service	bet. Pacific/ Dean Sreets
Pan-Asian	718-858-3880
All cards	Mon-Thu 11:30am-11pm Fri- &
Beer, wine & sake	F, Sat 11:30am-11:30pm
www.wildgingervegan.com	Sun 12pm-11pm

For description, see under Soho.

 Indicates we especially recommend this restaurant for the quality of the food

QUEENS

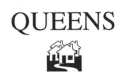

ANNAM BRAHMA [v] $

Full service
Indian vegetarian
$4.00-12.00 (all cards)
No alcohol

84-43 164th Street
at Hillside Avenue
718-523-2600
M-Tu,Th-Sa 11am-10pm
W 11am-4pm; Su 12-10pm

This year marks the fortieth anniversary of Annam Brahma, [They opened in 1971.],, making it one of the most venerable vegetarian restaurants in the city. It was started and is currently operated by followers of the spiritual leader Sri Chimnoy, who encourages his pupils to observe a vegetarian diet, to meditate and to give something back to the community. (Pictures of Chimnoy running marathons and striking poses festoon the walls). His pupils founded this restaurant to contribute to the common weal; and the high quality of the food bespeaks their dedication to higher principles. Particularly recommended are the delicious Chapati Roll-Ups that are stuffed with either an American Veggie Burger filling or an Indian Curry filling, and the Veggie Kebabs made with soy meat.

BUDDHA BODAI [v] $

Full service
Chinese (kosher)
$7.95-14.95 (all cards)
No alcohol.

42-96 Main Street
at Cherry Avenue
718-939-1188
daily 11am-11pm

There is a wide array of dishes to choose from--Veg. Snail to Sweet and Sour Fish. Indeed, the range of ersatz is so exhaustive that it put us in mind of those Taoist temple kitchens in which chefs flaunt their ingenuity by creating ever more elaborate mock meat dishes. But we did not enjoy our dining experience here; mainly because the manager was brusque and discourteous and refused to entertain any questions as to which dishes were vegan and which were not.

DOSA HUTT [v] $

Counter service
South Indian Vegetarian
$3.00-8.00 (no cards)
No alcohol

45-63 Bowne Street
(Flushing)
718-961-5897
daily 10am-9pm

This is India's answer to the Pizza Hut. Dosas, which are enormous crepes filled with spicy potato mixtures, do bear a resemblance to pizza, but I'll take a dosa over a pizza any time. The dosas here are tip-top, We especially relished the Masala Dosa. As with Dossa Diner, they're biigger and cheaper here than in the Big Dosa!

HAPPY BUDDHA [ve] $

Full service
Chinese
All major cards
No alcohol
www.happybuddha.com

135-37 37th Avenue
(Flushing)
718-358-0079
daily 11am-10pm

There are a myriad of tasty dishes on the menu that would make the Buddha and any other vegan very happy indeed. The vegetarian mock duck was a personal favorite.

MAHARAJAH QUALITY [v] $
SWEETS & SNACKS

Full service
International vegetarian
All Cards
No alcohol

73-10 37th Avenue
bet. 73rd/ 74th Streets
718-505-2680
daily 10am-10pm

As with Shamiana, this is Indian cuisine at its most caseous. The sweets and the dishes in the back are awash in milk, yogurt, cream, ghee, butter and cheese. You can pick your way through the menu to find vegan dishes, but is it really worth it?

NATURE & OEGANIC LIFE CAFÉ [v] $

Counter service
Chinese-Japanese-American fusion, organic
M, V
No alcohol
www. Breadaorganic.com

41-46 College Point Boulevard
bet. 41st Road/ Sanford
718-886-1888
daily 8:30am-8pm

Brenda Hwang, the proprietor of this cozy little café in Queens is a former fashion designer, an alumna of FIT, who had her own boutique on Fifth Avenue, and a staff of forty people toiling

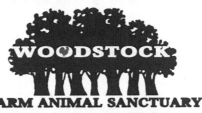
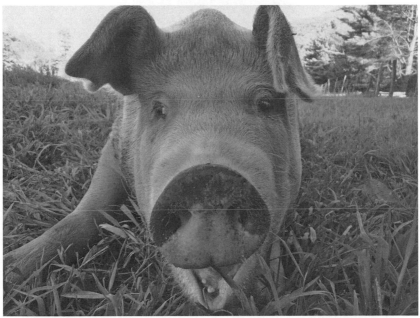

under her. In 2006, she turned her back on her thriving design company, and opened this vegetarian café-cum-bakery, which serves delicious and healthful vegetarian food, fusing Japanese, Chinese, and American cuisines.

The cafe and bakery are on the site of her former design studio in which she turned out the dress designs that made her one of the world's top Chinese-American fashion designers. As befits such a gifted artisan, the interior is elegantly designed, and the walls are adorned with her hand-painted murals and sumi-e paintings. But why, we wondered, did she give up such an enviable career?

Nonplussed, we overcame our reticence and asked her why she would have forsaken her successful fashion-designing business to become a full-time baker, chef, and restaurant owner. She told us that as a devout Buddhist she felt a special calling, actuated by the first precept of *ahimsa,* to try to help enlighten the public by purveying healthful vegetarian food and providing them with instruction on how to prepare it. To that end, she offers free cooking classes every fourth Thursday of the month.

We started with Wonton with Spicy Sauce which was piquant and bracing. Then we had The Dragon Roll Avocado, The New York Roll, and the Hawaiian Roll. They each contained an exotic mixture of ingredients that bewitched the palate. These dishes were followed by Pan Fried Rice Noodles with Vegetables; followed by Eggplant with String Beans and Basil, plus a Vegetable Medley that was held together with a lettuce wrap—three entrees that had the savory goodness of home-cooked food. That same wholesome savoriness characterized all the other dishes we tried—including that chestnut of Chinese menus--Vegan General Tsao's Chicken done up in a healthful manner with minimal use of salt and oil, and no MSG.

For dessert, we particularly relished the vegan Tiramisu. And the organic coffee, which is made with Kangen water—[That is, water that has been alkalinized by a special machine that was invented by a Japanese doctor, Dr. Kangen.]--was superb coffee, In fact we can say, without hyperbole, it is the best we've ever tasted. (Must have been the Kangen water?)

Most of her pastries are vegan, but a few, unaccountably, are made with eggs [Eggs are not Buddhist!]. No other animal ingredients were used in their preparation; so we were somewhat baffled by their incongruous presence on the menu. Otherwise, the food is totally vegan.

There is a healthful array of juices on offer. We imbibed the Celery, Carrot Apple tonic to our deep satisfaction.

Nature & Organic Life, is a must for those who love healthful vegetarian Chinese home-style cuisine.

ONENESS FOUNTAIN HEART [v] $$ 👍

	157-19 72md Avenue
Full service	(Flushing)
International vegetarian	718-591-3663
All cards)	daily 11:30-9pm
No alcohol	W 11:00-9:00

Yet another restaurant that is operated by disciples of Sri Chimnoy. In addition to the -blue facades that all the restaurants share, they also have in common an uncommon devotion to high culinary standards and service. The dishes to try here are the Duck Surprise, which is made with vegetarian mock duck, and the Vegetarian Meatloaf. My personal favorite was Thai Heaven, which consists of spicy tofu skin in a delicate coconut sauce. It's worth taking a cab from Manhattan for this one.

ORGANIC VILLAGE [ve] $ 👍

Counter service
Organic raw food café
Cash only
www.organicvillagenyc.com

79-15 Cooper Avenue
near 69th Drive (Glendale)
718-894-4369
M-Sa 10am-8pm; Su 10am-4pm

It's an arduous trek from Manhattan to Organic Village but for our money, it's well worth the puff that it takes to get out here. Organic Village owner, Ryan, and his raw food chef sister have created an oasis of vegan rawfoodism in this gritty industrial section of Queens where the standard fare is meat 'n' fries. The prices are moderate compared to those of the gaudier marts of rawfoodism in Manhattan, and the food bears comparison with the best of them. With its busts of the Buddha and Taoist accents, its well-lit interior is serene and relaxing. We sat at the bar—which commands a view of the spotless kitchen—and watched our food being prepared. While waiting, we lubricated ourselves with a Coconut-Berry Smoothie and a Blueberry Dream Smoothie. Both were pluperfect. It took a while for them to assemble our Taco Burrito and our Shitake Burger. But it was worth the wait. The Shitake Burger is the best veggie burger, raw or cooked, that we've tasted in eons Ditto for the Taco Burrito. For dessert, we relished their Chia Seed Pudding, as we did everything about this culinary diamond in the rough. *NB: OV has temporarily suspended their restaurant service; they are available for take out orders and deliveries only. They will also continue to provide hands-on instruction in the preparation of raw food—by appointment only.*

PANORAMA CAFE [v] $ 👍

86-14 Parsons Boulevard
(Jamaica)
Counter service
International vegetarian   718-526-0723
No cards   M-F 7am-9pm
No alcohol   Sa-Su 9am-8pm
www.Panoramacafe.org

This place may be suitable for the most lacto of lacto vegetarians, but it is far too caseous to be recommended for vegans. Unfortunately the dishes are overloaded with dairy and eggs (chick embryos.) While it is true that they offer Daiya cheese as a substitute, it is rather tedious to have to make substitutions for every dish. Although this is another of the Sri Chimnoy restaurants, and we would love to praise it, we could not find one vegan dish on the menu. We cannot give a favorable review to a restaurant that doesn't keep eggs and cheese to a minimum. This place is replete with them.

SMILE OF THE BEYOND [v] *$$* 👍

Counter service
International vegetarian
$4.00-6.00 (no cards)
No alcohol

86-14 Parsons Boulevard
(Jamaica)
718-739-7453
M-F 7am-4pm
Sa 7am-3pm

Not all restaurants in Queens are run by followers of Sri Chimnoy, it only seems that way. This astoundingly inexpensive luncheonette serves delicious veggie burgers, and generous salads that would cost the earth in a Manhattan eatery. All three Chimnoy places are worth the trek from Manhattan. At this place, so economical are the prices that the train fare will probably end up costing more than the meal!

VEGGIE CASTLE [ve] *$* 👍

Counter service
Caribbean
All cards
No alcohol

132-091 Liberty Avenue
near Van Wyck Expwy
718-641-8342
daily 10am-10pm

Last year Veggie Castle moved to Queens from its original location in Brooklyn, where it had struck a decided blow for veganism and animal rights by turning a White Castle fast food restaurant into a vegan Rasta restaurant. When Veggie Castle first opened, it was as though the farm animals had revolted and taken over the farm! The hostages had overpowered their captors!

Some enterprising vegetarian business folks had actually taken over a former burger joint and turned it into a vegetarian restaurant that serves the Veggie Castle Burger along with an array of delicious dishes that you won't find in your typical fast food place--such as Curried Soy Chicken, BBQ Soy Chunks With Pineapple, and ersatz Shepherd's Pie. We had a Spicy Black Bean Burger that was much the best veggie burger we'd ever tasted. We followed this with an order of Turmeric Bean Curd Duck that really showed off to advantage the culinary talent of Veggie Castle's Rasta *chefs de cuisine*. Instead of soda pop and shakes, Veggie Castle's juice bar serves a range of fresh fruit/vegetable juices and smoothies. Veggie Castle is giving fast food such a good name that, in the future, all burger joints may be dishing up Wheat Grass Juice and Veggie Burgers. It's cause for hope.

👍 Indicates we especially recommend this restaurant for the quality of the food

THE BRONX

H.I.M. [v] **$**

Counter service
Organic Caribbean
All Cards
No alcohol

754 Burke Avenue
Bronx
718-653-9627
daily 10am-9pm

The Bronx's first vegan restaurant is H.I.M. No, it's not a sexist cabal. H.I.M. is an acronym for His Imperial Highness, Hailie Selasie, the late emperor of Ethiopia who is regarded as the founding prophet of Rastafarianism. Rastafarians abstain from alcohol and all animal flesh. Pictures of Haile Selassie and other famous Rastafarians festoon the walls. Nazar, the Antiguan native who owns H.I.M., is a very religious guy who infuses his food with ethereal flavors. The menu changes every day, but the dishes we sampled were all pretty tasty. Among them were the Rasta standards: Barbecued Vegi Chicken, Kalaloo, Scrambled Tofu, Tofu Balls, Yam and Tofu Stew. For dessert, we had a slice of Almond Cake and a Mango Turnover. From the outside, H.I.M. looks a bit unkempt, and from the inside it also looks unkempt, but the food is good. Whether you're a HIM or a HER, if you're a connoisseur of pretty good vegan food, you should hasten to H.I.M.

VEGAN'S DELIGHT [v] **$$**

Counter service
Organic Caribbean
All Cards
No alcohol

3565 Boston Road
at Tiemann Avenue
718-653-4140
M-Sa 8am-6:30pm

Like Healthy Pleasure and Imhoteps, in Queens and Brooklyn, respectively, Vegan's Delight is a combination health-food store and restaurant. Is it worth the trip from Manhattan to eat here? That depends: If you're a connoisseur of Ital food as we are, then the trip is certainly warranted. However, there are places in Manhattan and Brooklyn that do the Ital thing just as well if not better. For instance: The Uptown Juice Bar and Veggie Castle--to list but two. We savored the Curried Bean Curd, the Ital Stew, and the Eggplant Melange, and commend it to you.

WOODSTOCK

GARDEN CAFE [v] *$$* 👍

6 Old Forge Road
(on the Village Green)
845-679-3600
W-M 11:30am-9pm

Full service
Global Organic
All cards
Organic wines & beers

One of our favorite New York escapes is to spend the weekend in Woodstock. It is still redolent of the arts colony that it used to be in the early part of the last century, and of the hippie era of the sixties. Now we can augment the pleasure of our weekend getaways by dining at the Garden Café. It was opened four years ago by chef Pam Brown.

In addition to her regular lunch and dinner menus, daily specials include a Garden Bowl, consisting of greens, whole grains, vegetables, beans, tofu, tempeh, or seitan. We started with an autumnal salad of spinach with roasted pears and pecans with a cranberry dressing. *Extraordinare!*

Then we tucked into an international array of dishes that included Indian Vegetable and Chickpea Enchiladas, served with a Bombay Sauce, and a Curried Apple-Coconut Salad on the side. *Sensationel!* We tossed this off with multiple toasts of organic vegan wine and beer. We also had the Southwest Black Bean and Roasted Sweet Potato Burger with Guacamole Salsa and a wedge of Vegan Cheddar. *Magnifique!* After downing these, our faces beamed with satisfaction.

We had to bolt in order to be on time for a concert at the Maverick; so we skipped the Warm Chocolate Brownie with Hot Fudge Sauce, served with Vegan Whipped Cream, and the Raw Agave Pistachio Gelato. But we will be returning tomorrow night, [after we visit the Woodstock Farm Animal Sanctuary, and the Catskill Animal Sanctuary], to sit in reposeful ease under the poplar trees and gaze at the town square "thinking green thoughts in a green shade."

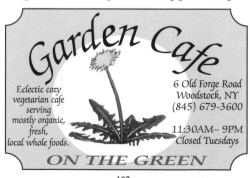

Garden Cafe

Eclectic cozy vegetarian cafe serving mostly organic, fresh, local whole foods.

6 Old Forge Road
Woodstock, NY
(845) 679-3600

11:30AM– 9PM
Closed Tuesdays

ON THE GREEN

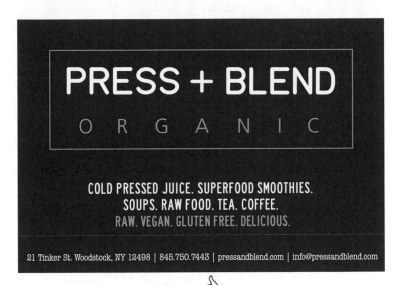

COLD PRESSED JUICE. SUPERFOOD SMOOTHIES.
SOUPS. RAW FOOD. TEA. COFFEE.
RAW. VEGAN. GLUTEN FREE. DELICIOUS.

21 Tinker St. Woodstock, NY 12498 | 845.750.7443 | pressandblend.com | info@pressandblend.com

PRESS + BLEND ORGANIC CAFE [v] *$$*

Counter service
Organic, raw, gluten free
All cards
Organic wines & beers
Pressandblend.com

21 Tinker Street
(at Rock City Road)
845-750-7443
W-M 10am-6pm

Upon stepping foot in Press + Blend--Woodstock's first Cold-Press Juice Bar—our first impression was of an elegantly apponted cafe with a bright, upbeat, cheerful atmosphere. When the friendly counter girl saw us staring fixedly at the attractive array of bottled juices in the cooler, she offered to enlighten us about them. Patiently, she explained that they were cold-press juices that had been produced by the legendary Norwalk Juicer. If they looked more vivid and potent than *jus ordinaire,* it's because they are. The Norwalk produces a juice that has 8-15 times the mineral and vitamin content than that of a rotary juicer. For this reason it has more staying power than a regular juicer, and may be bottled and refrigerated for up to three days. After drinking "Press # 7," we felt lighter on our feet and more acute mentally. We knew that we just had to come back for one of their superfood smoothies. Sure enough, after listening to a few customers extolling the merits of smoothies laced with gogiberries, maca, raw cacao, hemp seed, spirulina, and various other super foods from the menu, it made us want to try them all. The smoothie we ended up trying was "Blend # 1: The Secret to Happiness." And darned if it didn't seem to be just that ! A thrill of euphoria tingled through us as we left the store. However, as recovering choco-holics, we couldn't leave without snagging some raw vegan chocolates to fortify us for the drive to New York City....Now we have one more compelling reason for visiting Woodstock as often as possible!

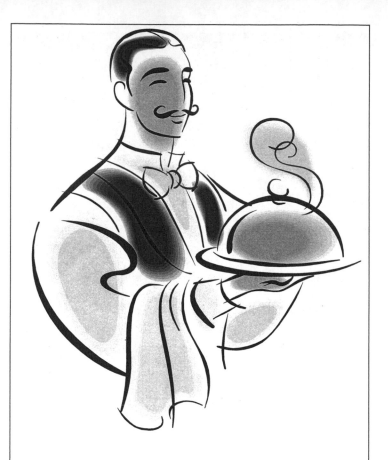

"The discovery of a new vegan restaurant dish does more for the well-being of the human race than the discovery of a new star."

...Jean Brillat Savarin (1756-1825)
[revised with apologies]

CYBERSPACE

VEGGIE BROTHERS.COM [ve] **$**

Shipped frozen to your door
Global vegan, organic
All Cards
No alcohol

www.veggiebrothers.com
in cyberspacce
1-877-VEGAN-55
daily 24hours

Chef Made Vegan Meals Delivered right to your door, anywhere in the USA & Canada, so you can enjoy this special "Vegan Cuisine for the Mainstream" anytime, anywhere. Now you have no excuse for not sticking to a vegan diet even in the remotest hinterlands. Veggie Brothers, the first online gourmet vegan restaurant features vegan versions of Americas favorite dishes that delight vegan and carnivores alike. Vegan athlete, holistic health expert and vegan food connoisseur, Michael Balducci, has whipped up a brand new website that demonstrates a commitment not just to plant based guilt-free indulgences, but a commitment to animal welfare, environmentalism, and vegan nutritional education.

Just place your order online and products are shipped via UPS and arrive conveniently at the destination of your choice. Reheating was so easy and the taste so fresh, it will seem like a top gourmet vegan chef was just in your kitchen. Choose from a delicious array of now over 100 healthful chef-crafted options that includes entrees, soups, appetizers, and decadent desserts. We tried the vegan Beef Wellington, and vegan Chicken Pot Pie and fancied that we were in one of the world's great vegan restaurants in Manhattan Candle 79, Franchia, Caravan of Dreams, in Manhattan, or Vegethus in Sao Paulo. We also savored their Manchurian Pepper Steak (with a side of brown rice). It was on sale as a daily special. Made from seitan, it was so artfully prepared that we had the illusion of dining at Zen Palate Only the glare of the flashing neon light reminded us that we were stopping for two nights at a Red Roof Inn, a thousand miles from the nearest vegan restaurant.

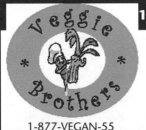

TOP TEN JUICE BARS

Ö

Although they don't yet outnumber the alcohol bars, or the coffee bars, juice bars are starting to crop up all over town. Unhappily, many of them--like Gray's Papaya--serve meat along with their smoothies and juices. [Recently, we had to drop Juice Generation for serving chicken sandwiches,, and Liquetira for serving tuna fish sandwices.] So we picked places that serve only vegan dishes to go with their drinks. Not so long ago, New Yorkers used to start the day with a shot of bourbon or a mug of java; now, as like as not, they'll get their hearts started with a shot of "green plasma"--wheat grass juice, brimming with enzymes, antioxidants, chlorophyll, and phytonutrients.

THE JUICE PRESS [ve]   at 3 locations: JP 1
70 East 1st Street
bet. 1st / 2nd Avenues

JP2
279 East 10th Street
bet. 1st / A Avenues

JP 3
1050 3rd Avenue
At 62nd Street
8am-8pm

The standard by which all others are measured. The best smoothies in the universe! This is the only juice bar in the city that uses 100% organic, fresh fruits and juices.

Juice Press's criteria for hygiene and service are exacting. Working surfaces and equipment are constantly being scrubbed with an unsleeping vigilance. Well-mannered, eager-to-please, and efficient, his staff clearly love their work.

The Juice Press uses a Norwalk hydraulic press. (Up to five times more of the enzymes, minerals and vitamins are expressed in the juices by this method than by any other.) For a bracing sandwich, try JP' Schmear homemade vegan rosemary cream cheese and marinated cucumbers on a toasted sprouted grain bagel. . For a Smoothie, try the Rain Forest a refreshing blend of lemon, mint, coconut water, banana, and other tropical ingredients They're a ticket to esophageal paradise.

.GREEN PIRATE[v]   Grand Army Plaza Farmers' Market
Prospect Park West / Union Ave.
Sa 8:30 am - 5 pm
[April-November]

Green Pirate is the only juice-truck of its kind in the country. Founded and operated by Deborah Smith, a graduate of the Institute for Integrative Nutrition, Green Pirate is dedicated to improving the quality of life and health of the community.

From the Pirate truck, which runs on bio-diesel, Deborah dispenses such exotic juice combinations as the Cantaloupe Creamsicle (canteloupe, carrot, orange juice and coconut milk); and Hot Pink Limeade (red apple, lemon, lime, cucumber, and sweet beet). She also sells fresh green coconut water. If you miss her at her Farmers' market location in Park Slope on Saturday; you can find her at the flea-market in DUMBO from 11am-5pm on Sundays. During the winter months Deborah proffers nutritional counseling. She can be reached at Deborah@greenpirate.com

RAWVOLUTION [ve]

504 East 12th Street
bet. Avenues A / B
daily 10:am-10pm

This raw food delicatessen-cum-juice bar offers a range of juices and juice combinations along with raw entrées like the Big Matt Burger, and Indonesian Kelp Noodles. Try their Green Juice and their Vanilla Mint Lemonade,

PERELANDRA [v] $

175 Remsen Street
bet. Court/ Clinton
718-855-6068
M-F 8:30-8:30
Sa 9:30-8:30:
Su 11-7

For the post prandial beverage, we sipped their Avocado Smoothie. Which contains Coconut Juice, Avocado, Agave Nectar, and Fresh Lime Juice. We specifically requested that they make it with agave nectar as they ordinarily make it with honey.

GREENER PASTURES [ve]

Union Square Greenmarket
16th St. / Union Square West
M,W, F, Sa 8am-7pm

On Mondays, Wednesdays, Fridays and Saturdays of every week, Stewart, the proprietor, serves up wheat grass juice and effervescent good humor to the patrons who mob his stand. They swear he has the sweetest grass in the city. A one ounce shot is $3.00 a double shot is $5.00. ;Recently; Stewart enlarged his repertoire of hices. He now offers a green juice combination, which consists of pea sprouts , sunflower spouts, carrots, apples, and ginger. The spouts are grown by Stewart at his indoor farm in Brooklyn; but the carrots, apples, and ginger are supplied by other farmers in the market; so their freshness and quality are guaranteed. This drink, served in capacious containers. The small is $5; the large is $7/. Stewart also sells flats of Wheat Grass as well as succulent salad greens.

UPTOWN JUICE BAR [ve]

54 West 125th Street
daily 8am-10pm

They offer a wide array of juices and juice combinations that are designed to cure everything from asthma to impotence. The fruit smoothes are delicious, and the Caribbean style vegan food is first rate.

FOOD SHOPPING

It's possible to eat cheaply in New York. It's also possible to spend your life savings on a single meal (though much easier for meat-eaters than for vegans!). This applies to restaurants as well as to shops, which range from the most luxurious importers to inexpensive, dependable local farm products. Below are some notable places that won't break your budget; for obvious reasons, this is not a comprehensive list. Individual addresses are listed on the following page.

SUPERMARKETS

these, and it The largest stores carry health food items, soy milk, and the like, but their prices are not usually any lower than large health food shops for these goods. The New York chains, listed in roughly ascending order of price (quality is quite similar): Associated, Sloan's, Gristede's, Met Food, D'Agostino, Food Emporium, WholeFoods.

PRODUCE

There are greenmarkets, also called farmer's markets, on certain days in public squares, where producers drive truckloads of fresh and often organic fruits and vegetables into the city from their farms in upstate New York, Pennsylvania, and New Jersey. The prices and quality can't be beat, and there's a festive atmosphere to these events. Of course, you'll find only what's in season, so there are slim pickings during the cold winter months. Union Square is the largest of boasts a vegan bakery stall called Body & Soul with great treats both sweet and savory.

The next choice for organic produce is shopping at a large health food store like Wholesome Market, Integral Yoga or Commodities. Prices are a bit higher, but the quality is excellent.

For non-organic produce, the Asian shops along Canal Street in Chinatown and on First Avenue around 7th Street in the East Village have the lowest prices. Otherwise, supermarkets and the 24-hour groceries that line many New York streets are fairly reliable.

BULK GOODS, SPICES, ETC.

The larger health food shops all have a section where you can buy grains, beans, nuts, dried fruit, flour and snacks in bulk, most of it organic. For non-organic bulk goods and wonderful spices at low prices, try the Indian shops around Lexington and 28th Street or First Avenue and 6th Street.

BOOKS BY RYNN BERRY

FAMOUS VEGETARIANS
and their favorite recipes

Lives and Lore from Buddha to the Beatles

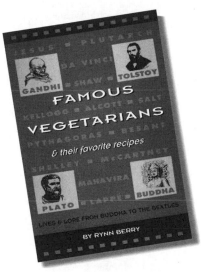

"Berry writes beautifully, with a genuine gustatory relish for words and savory asides. The recipes are delightful...many researched and translated for the first time." —*The Boston Book Review*

"Scholarship at the end of a fork—and for writing it Berry deserves an 'A'."
—*Vegetarian Times*

"Entertaining and educational..."
—*Vegetarian Voice*

"Impeccably researched and written."
—*The Animals' Agenda*

"The 70 recipes are not only fascinating, but have been kitchen-tested by the author for savoriness..." —*Yoga Journal*

292 pages   **$15.95** *paperback*

Copy this form to order books. Other books by Rynn Berry on reverse side.

✂ ---

PYTHAGOREAN PUBLISHERS / P.O. Box 8174 / New York, NY 10116

—— copies *Famous Vegetarians & Their Favorite Recipes* @ $15.95	$ ——
—— copies *The New Vegetarians* @ $10.95	$ ——
—— copies *Food for the Gods* @ $19.95	$ ——

Add postage: $3.00 for one book, $1.00 for each additional book $ ——

TOTAL ENCLOSED $ ——

NAME _____

ADDRESS _____

CITY _____ STATE/ZIP_____ PHONE _____

FAVORITE SHOPS

<u>HARLEM</u>

FAIRWAY FRUITS & VEGETABLES
Huge produce and natural food store.

2328 Twelfth Avenue
at West 132nd Street

7 GRAINS HEALTH FOODS
Health food shop.

2259 Seventh Avenue
at 133rd Street

<u>UPPER WEST SIDE</u>

GARY NULL'S UPTOWN WHOLEFOODS

2307 Broadway
at West 89th Street

Health food grocery with bustling juice bar and kosher vegetarian salad bar.

HEALTH NUTS
Health food shop with juice bar.

2611 Broadway
at West 99th Street

WHOLEFOODS MARKET
Organic supermarket.

10 Columbus Circle
at 60th Street

<u>UPPER EAST SIDE</u>

HEALTH NUTS
Health food shop with juice bar.

1208 Second Avenue
bet. 63rd/64th Streets

MATTER OF HEALTH
health food shop with juice bar.

1478 First Avenue
at 77th Street

NATURAL FRONTIER
Organic grocery with emphasis on vegetarian and vegan.

1424 Third Avenue
at 81st Street

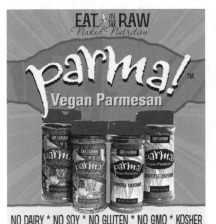
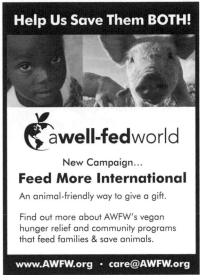
<u>MIDTOWN WEST</u>

HEALTHY CHELSEA
Health food shop with juice bar.

248 West 23rd Street
bet. Seventh/Eighth Avenues

NICE N' NATURAL
Health food shop with juice bar.

673 Ninth Avenue
bet. 46th / 47th Streets

ORGANIC MARKET
Health food shop.

229 Seventh Avenue
bet. 23rd/24th Streets

SIVANANDA YOGA VEDANTA CENTER
Exercise, breathing, relaxation, diet, and mediation

243 West 24th Street
bet. 7th/8th Avenues

WESTERLY NATURAL MARKET
Well stocked organic grocery.

911 Eighth Avenue
at 54th Street

WHOLEFOODS MARKET
Organic supermarket.

250 Seventh Avenue
at 24th Street

BETH'S FARM KITCHEN
Jams, jellies and pickled vegetables F, Sa year-round.

Union Square Greenmarket
bet. 17th St / Union Sq.West

BODY & SOUL
All-vegan baked goods stand.M F year-round.

Union Square Greenmarket
bet. 17th St / Union Sq.West

FANTASY FRUIT FARM
Blueberries, strawberries, raspberries, seedless grapes
Saturdays, June-Nov.

Union Square Greenmarket
bet. 17th St. / Union Sq. West

FOODS OF INDIA
Another Indian grocery.

121 Lexington Avenue
bet. 29th/30th Streets

HEALTH NUTS
Well-provisioned health food store.

835 2nd Avenue
bet. 44th/ 45th Streets

KALUSTYAN

123 Lexington Avenue
bet. 28th / 29th Streets

Well-stocked Indian Grocery. They feature bulk items such as raw pistachio nuts and sun-dried strawberries.

KEITH'S FARM
Heirloom herbs, garlics and greens, We Sa, Ju -Nov.

Union Square Greenmarket
bet. 17th St. / Union Sq. West

LOCUST GROVE FRUIT FARM
A cornucopia of delicious fruit, W, Sa year-round.

Union Square Greenmarket
bet. 17th St. / Union Sq. West

OLIVIERS & CO
Olive oil merchants

Grand Central Terminal
near Track 17

This store specializes in premium olive oils from all the Mediterranean countries plus Uruguay. They also sell a highly addictive sun-dried tomato powder for sprinkling on salads and suchlike vegan fare.

PHILLIPS FARMS
:

Union Square Greenmarket
bet. 17th/ Union Sq. West

Peaches, Raspberries, Blueberries and Blackberries. March-December, M, Sa 8am-6pm.

RICK'S PICKS

Union Square Greenmarket
bet. 17th/ Union Sq. West

Rick, an Andover and Yale alum, quit his job as PBS producer to become a picklemeister. Favorite pickle is Wasabean (green beans and wasabi). Wednesdays sunrise to sunset, year round.

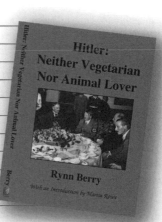

TRADER JOE'S
142 East 14th Street
at Union Sq. East
An offbeat supermarket, Joe's is famous for its unusual and inexpensive products, like wild blueberry juice, dark chocolate-covered espresso beans, and, our favorite, chili-spiced dried mango slices.

WINDFALL FARM
Union Square Greenmarket
Wide range of organic greens, We, Sa year round
bet. 17th St. / Union Sq. West

GREENWICH VILLAGE

INTEGRAL YOGA NATURAL FOODS
229 West 13th Street
Health food shop
bet. Seventh/Eighth Avenues
Good quality and price on organics and bulk goods, plus hot and cold buffet. Some raw food dishes. Very popular.

LIFETHYME
410 Sixth Avenue
at Eighth Street
One-stop shopping for large selection of exclusively organic produce, bulk goods, vitamins, herbal nostrums, and cruelty-free cosmetics. Amazing salad bar and delicious vegetarian food to go. Their vegan bakery turns out scrumptious pastries and prides itself on not using milk eggs or cheese in any of their cakes cookies or pies. They have a spiffy juice bar, and a good selection of books on nutrition and healing. Recently, they've added a living foods section with delicious raw pies, cakes and entrees.

NY ARTIFICIAL

13 8th Avenue
At West 12th Street
Handbags, jewelry, accessories,, shoes, apparel, and makeup.
www. nyartificial.com • 646-340-0442 • 646-340-0813

ORGANIC AVENUE-2
43 8th Avenue
bet. Jane / Horatio Streets
Hemp and organic clothing, organic lifestyle products, fresh, raw and organic produce collective.

STELLA McCARTNEY
429 West 14th Street
bet. 9th/ 10th Avenues
The scion of Sir Paul sells vegan shoes and cruelty-free clothing of her own design.

PYTHAGOREAN PUBLISHERS

P.O. Box 8174, JAF Station, New York, NY 10116 Tel./Fax: 718-622-8002

Rynn Berry

Food for the Gods

Vegetarianism & the World's Religions

384 pages 0-9626169-2-3 $19.95 paperback

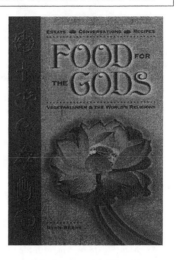

"*Food for the Gods* is eloquently philosophical; it is eavesdropping on the erudite."—**Dr. Kristin Aronson**, Professor of Philosophy, Western Connecticut University

"Rynn Berry has created a memorable feast for mind, body, and soul. *Food for the Gods* makes a tasty and terrific gift for the cook who has everything, including a lively curiosity and an adventurous culinary spirit."—**Lorna Sass**, author of *Lorna Sass' Complete Vegetarian Kitchen*

"The aptly named Rynn Berry has become the official vegan ambassador. His books treat vegetarianism not merely as a cult but as a culture. For Berry, the act of eating is not just a matter of sustenance, it's also a novel and even a spiritual act. His latest, *Food for the Gods*, is a fascinating investigation into the world's great religions. Berry provides illuminating essays on vegetarianism in Jainism, Hinduism, Buddhism, Sufism, and other non-Western religions, as well as Christianity and Judaism. He interviews religious thinkers who are also vegetarians, and he supplies recipes for dishes that have come from these different cultures. The result is a banquet for the taste buds of the mind."—**Jack Kroll**, Senior Editor *Newsweek*

Rynn Berry is the historical advisor to the North American Vegetarian Society and the author of *The New Vegetarians* and *Famous Vegetarians and Their Favorite Recipes*, a biographical history of vegetarianism that ranges from Pythagoras and the Buddha through to Isaac Bashevis Singer and the Beatles. He lives in Brooklyn.

Also by Rynn Berry:
Famous Vegetarians and Their Favorite Recipes: Lives and Lore from the Buddha to the Beatles
The New Vegetarians

COMMODITIES EAST   165 First Avenue
                                              at 10th Street
Health food shop with good quality and prices on organic produce and bulk goods.

4TH STREET FOOD COOP   58 East Fourth Street
                                              bet. Bowery and Second
All produce from leafy greens to tubers is organic, and the granola, grains, nuts and other bulk
times are mostly so. Non-members are welcome.

HEALTHFULY OEGANIC MARKET   98 East Fourth Street
                                              bet. 1st / 2nd Avenues
Healthfully carries a full range of raw, vegan, gluten-free foods, organic products, and groceries
as well as natural health and beauty aids. They specialize in raw, organic whole food vitamins;
fully handcrafted organic herbal extracts ns supplements. They frequently have sales on premium
health food products such as Zico Coconut water, etc.

HIGH VIBE HEALTH & HEALING   138 East Third Street (rear)
                                              bet. 1st / A Avenues
A raw food superstore since '93 created by Bob Dagger, who has collected and created some of
the largest selections of rawfood snacks, food, supplements, super foods, appliances, potions,
books, beauty care, along with his nutritional counseling and classes; your one stop for
everything you need for better health. A must visit also on line for great free recipes and free
information: highvibe.com.

INDIA SPICE HOUSE   99 First Avenue
Indian grocery, 24 hours   at 6th Street
Smaller than the Lexington stores, and the foodstuffs don't move so quickly, but still good—
especially if you need some fenugreek or asafoetida in the middle of the night. 400 kinds of beer.

JIVAMUKTI YOGA CENTER   841 Broadway
                                              bet. 13th/ 14th Streets
Yoga Center and emporium that sells yoga paraphernalia, eco-friendly clothing, books. It also
features a new vegan cafe -cum-juice bar called JivamukTea, Try the Raw Lasagna, the Creator
BLT, and chef Matthew Kenney's delicious raw desserts.

LIVE LIVE & ORGANIC   261 East 10th Street
                                              bet. 1st Avenue / Avenue A
Raw foods boutique, featuring, a wide selection of books, super foods, snacks, potions,
energizers and rejuvenatives. Also on sale are dehydrators, juicers and other accouterments of
the raw food lifestyle. Consult their website: www.live-live.com

SUSTAINABLE NYC 139 Avenue A
bet. 9th/ 10th Streets
Local, organic, re-cycled, fair-trade, re-purposed, biodegradable, products and gifts.

WHOLEFOODS UNION SQUARE 40 East 14th Street
Organic supermarket. at Broadw

SOHO

BABY CAKES 240 Broome Street
Vegan baked goods. bet. Orchard/ Ludlow Streets

EKOVARUHUSET 123 Ludlow Street
Organic, fair trade clothing

EARTH MATTERS 177 Ludlow Street
Organic market with salad bar bet. Stanton/ Houston

GUSS'S LOWER EAST SIDE PICKLES 85-87 Orchard Street
bet. Broome/ Grand
Pickled tomatoes, artichoke hearts as well the old standbys. This shop and its owner starred in
the motion picture Crossing Delancey Street.

MAY WAH HEALTHY VEG. FOOD 213 Hester Street
bet. Centre / Baxter
Chinese Vegetarian grocery store. Well-stocked with mock meats such as mock shrimp, mock
duck, mock squid, etc.

MOO SHOES 78 Orchard Street
bet. Grand/ Broome/ Streets
The best selection of cruelty-free shoes and accessories in the country.

OBSESSIVE COMPULSIVE COSMETICS
174 Lullow Street
bet. Houston / Stanton Streets
100% vegan cruelty free cosmetics and accessories in a stunning new bourtique.

ORGANIC AVENUE 156m Sullivan Street
Bet. W, Houston / Prince Streets
ORGANIC AVENUE 116 Suffolk Street
bet. Riivington / Delancey
Hemp and organic clothing, organic lifestyle products, fresh, raw and organic produce collective.

WHOLEFOODS MARKET 95 East Houston Street
Organic supermarket. at Bowery

BELL BATES
Large Health Food Grocery Store

97 Reade Street
bet. W.Bway / Church

COMMODITIES NATURAL FOODS MARKET
Vast health food shop with good bulk prices.

117 Hudson Street
at North Moore Street

WHOLEFOODS MARKET
Organic Supermarket

270 Greenwich Street

BROOKLYN

BACK TO THE LAND

142 Seventh Avenue
bet. Carroll Street/Garfield Place

Organically grown produce as well as grains, nuts and dried fruits are on offer. A wide range of books, magazines and tapes are for sale. There is a section for homeopathic remedies. And a well-stocked macro-biotic section.

DOWNTOWN NATURAL MARKET
Organic produce, Juice and Salad bars.

51 Willoughby Street
off Jay Street

FAIRWAY
The Manhattan food bazaar has come to Brooklyn.

480-500 Van Brunt Street
Red Hook

FLATBUSH FOOD COOP

1318 Corydon Road
bet.Rugby and Argyle Rds.

Fresh organic produce. Earth-friendly household products. Open to non-members

PARK SLOPE FOOD COOP
Members only organic market
Members pay 20% above cost. Closed to Non-members.

782 Union Street
bet. 6th & 7th Avenues

PERELANDRA NATURAL FOOD CENTER

175 Ramsen Street
at Court Street

Largest health food store in Brooklyn. Excellent juice bar and book section.

THE GARDEN
Well-stocked health food shop.

921 Manhattan Avenue
at Kent Street (Willamsburg)

GNOSIS CHOCOLATE (raw vegan chocolate)　　　40-03 27th Street
　　　　　　　　　　　　　　　　　　　　　　　Long Island City
[Available at Westerly, High Vibe, Live Live & Organic, Jivamukti Yoga, & WholeFoods]

NEIL'S NATURAL MARKET　　　　　　　　　46-10 Hollis Court Avneue
　　　　　　　　　　　　　　　　　　　　　　　(Flushing)
Organic produce, vitamins, rawfooods, herbs, homeopathy, cruelty-free body care products, and bulk items.

QUEENS HEALTH EMPORIUM　　　　　　　159-01 Horace Harding
Expy.Macrobiotic products, organic produce, juice bar.　　　(Flushing Meadows).

GOOD 'N' NATURAL　　　　　　　　　　　2173 White Plains Road
Exceptionally well stocked Health Food Store　　(bet. Pelham Pkwy/Lydig Ave)

MICAH PUBLICATIONS

THE SOURCE FOR JEWISH VEGETARIAN AND ANIMAL RIGHTS BOOKS

VEGAN COOKBOOKS WITH JEWISH TRADITION

www. micahbooks.com

RAW FOOD RESOURCES

New York has not only the greatest wealth of vegan and vegetarian restaurants in the world, it also has the greatest wealth of rawfood resources. If you count, Caravan of Dreams, Bonobos, and the Westerley Raw Food Bar, New York now boasts fourteen raw food restaurants, and a growing number of raw food boutiques like High Vibe and Live Live, where the aspiring rawfooder may obtain nutritional guidance, instruction on raw food preparation, raw food snacks and useful gadgets like Food Processors, Saladacos (spiralizers). dehydrators, et al.

Restaurants

Bonobos
Full raw menu

18 East 23rd Street
bet. Park Avenue/Broadway

Caravan of Dreams
Partial raw menu

405 East 6th Street

Juice Press, The   at 3 locations:

JP 1
70 East 1st Street
et. 1st / 2nd Avenues
JP2
279 East 10th Street
bet. 1st / A Avenues
JP 3
1050 3rd Avenue
At 62nd Street
8am-8pm

Organic vegan raw juices, smoothies, and food

Organic Avenue

116 Suffok Street
bet. Rivington/ Delancey Streets

Salads, raw dishes, and smoothies are prepared in the basement, and kept in a refrigerated display case on the ground floor.

Oganic Village
Organic raw food cafe

79-15 Cooper Avenue
near 69th Dr (Glendale)

Deliveries and raw food preparation classes only.

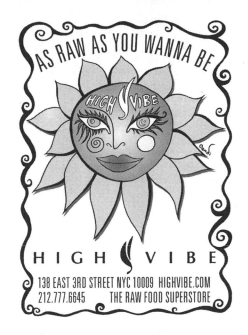
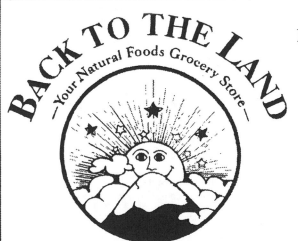

Pure Food and Wine
The ne plus ultra of raw food restaurants

54 Irving Place
bet. 17th/ 18th Streets

Pure Juice and Take Away
The take-out editon of Pure Food and Wine

125 1/2 East 17th Street
bet. 3rd Avenue / Irving Place

Quintessence
Mainly raw menu

263 East 10th Street
bet 1st Avenue / Avenue A

RAWvolution
All raw menu (Our current favorite.)

504 East 12th Street
bet. Avenues A / B

Raw Star
Full raw menu with juices and smoothies

687 Washington Avenue
at Prsspect Place
(Brooklyn)

Rockin' Raw
Full raw menu

78 N. Eighth St.
bet. Bedford / Driggs Avenues
(Brooklyn)

Westerly Raw Food Bar
Raw food deli in NW corner of the store

911 Eighth Avenue
at 54th Street

Raw Boutiques

Raw boutiques hold lectures, food prep classes; and sell super foods, raw snacks, books, gadgets, cosmetics, and other adjuncts of the vegan rawfood lifestyle.

BONOBOS REAL FOOD STORE
212-505-1200

18 East 23rd Street
bet. Park Avenue/ Broadway

HIGH VIBE
212-777-6645

138 East 3rd Street
bet. First / A Avenues

LIVE LIVE & ORGANIC
212-505-5504

261 East 10th Street
bet. 1st Avenue /Avenue A

ORGANIC AVENUE
212-334-4593

116 Suffok Street
bet. Rivington/ Delancey Streets

Raw Vegan Chocolate

GNOSIS CHOCOLATE

Available at Westerly, High Vibe,
Live Live & Organic, Jivamukti Yoga, et al.

Raw Potluck

HALLELUJAH ACRES POTLUCK   Last Sunday 484 West 43rs Street
212-594-0718   Apt. 34k (Rev. Lawrence Rush)

Hands On Raw Food Preparation Classes

LIVE LIVE & ORGANIC   212-505-5504

ORGANIC AVENUE   212-334-4593

ORGANIC VILLAGE   718-894-4369

QUINTESSENCE   212- 501-9700

RAW STAR   718-975-0304

Raw Foods on the Internet

HIGH VIBE   www. highvibe. com

LIVE- LIVE & ORGANIC   www.live-live.com

LIVING FOODS INSTITUTE   www.livingfoodsinstitute.com

HALLELUJAH ACRES   www. hacres.com

FRESH NETWORK   www. fresh-network.com

RAW NUTRTIONAL COUNSELING,   www. doctorgraham.cc

Raw Resorts
Ann Wigmore Natural Health Institute, PO Box 429, Rincon, PR 00677; (787) 868-6307.
Aris La Tham's SunJoy Natural Life Retreat, Coyaba Springs, River Gardens & Falls, Shaw
Park Ridge Estate, Ocho Rios, Jamaica (876) 441-0124, Sunfirefood@hotmail.com.
Vegan Living Foods Health Spa-Hippocrates Health Institute, 1441 Palmdale Court
West Palm Breach, FL 33411; (407) 471-8876
Vegan Health Spa-The Regency Health Spa, 2000 South Ocean Avenue, Hallandale,
FL 33009, (800) 454-0003
Water Fasting Center: True North, 4310 Lichau Road, Penngrove, CA 94951; (707) 792-2325

Guest Editorial

Oink! oink! Did you know that humans are omnivorous creatures more similar to pigs than we are to other animals? We both consume the largest variety of things available, natural or not, and derive some form of nourishment from whatever possible; however, few creatures can do what humans can with food! Just because we can eat almost anything doesn't mean we should. If optimal health is what you are seeking, then a diet of twinkies, cracker jacks, and cigarettes will not serve you well. Sure, everyone has an uncle that lived 100 years on whiskey and donuts. Science can easily explain him. Most of us would grow very sickly on that type of innutrition; not to mention your face would look like lizard's skin before your 50th birthday! Your vital forces would also be smothered by the consumption of such "garbage." These vital forces include creativity and spiritual happiness.

A preponderance of the world's population has been meeting their early demise due to illnesses that originate in the gut. People who live on concentrated synthetic foods are likely to end up on powerful synthetic medicines later in life. Contrary to what you might think your genes do not control your health and destiny. Rather, diet and lifestyle control how your genes will express themselves. This theory of genetic expression is cutting edge.

Diet includes not only the food you eat but also every thought and feeling you entertain. Feelings and thoughts feed your body cell by cell. Conversely, they can deprive, deplete, or inhibit your body's healing mechanisms. Unlike other animals, humans are the only creatures that have the capacity to either lower or raise their consciousness. We lower our consciousness, without full awareness, by deliberately poisoning ourselves with processed foods and other poor nutritional choices.

In conclusion, transcending to a higher conscious state and achieving remarkable physical, emotional and spiritual well being is just a few raw salads and juices away. Leave out all processed foods, poor food combinations, over-eating, and negative thinking. Instead, jump start your diet with a juice cleanse and/or a raw food cleanse. Remember, if you eat clean, you'll feel clean and be clear. *by Marcus Antebi , co-founder of The Juice Press (with contributions by Dr. Fred Bisci (author of Your Healthy Journey).*

ORIGINAL OUTSPOKEN ORGANIC

Angelica Kitchen

Regional Vegan Cuisine

300 E 12 St NYC

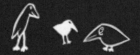

www.angelicakitchen.com

New York is the national capital of the publishing world, and is full of bookstores of all types—large chains carrying bestsellers, small dusty used bookshops, specialized technical or foreign-language stores. Here are some of our hangouts.

ALABASTER BOOKS.. 122 Fourth Avenue
Tel. 212- 982-3550 · at 12th
BOOKCOURT.. ..... 363 Court Street
Tel. 718-875-3677 bet. Pacific/Dean
BOOKCULTURE.. .. 336 W. 112 Street
Tel. 212-865-1588 at Broadway
BLUESTOCKINGS.. 172 Allen Street
Tel. 212-777-6028 bet. Stanton/Rivington Streets
CRAWFORD-DOYLE.. 1082 Madison Avenue
Tel. 212-288-6300 at 82nd Street
KITCHEN ARTS & LETTERS....................... 1435 Lexington
Tel. 212- 876-5550 at 94th Street
LOGOS BOOKS.................................... .... 1575 York Avenue
Tel. 212-517-7292 bet. 83rd/ *4th Streets
MERCER STREET BOOKS................................. 206 Mercer Street
Tel. 212-505-8615 at Bleecker Street
OPEN CENTER BOOKSTORE....................................... 22 E 30th St
Tel. 212) 219-2527. Ext. 108 bet. Madison/ Fifth Avenues
QUEST BOOKSHOP....................................... 240 East 53rd Street
Tel. 212- 758-5521 bet. Second/Third Avenues
SHAKESPEARE & CO.............................. .... 716 Broadway
Tel. 212-529-1330 at Waverly Place
ST. MARK'S BOOKSHOP...................................... 31 Third Avenue
Tel. 212-260-0443 at 9th Street
SPOONBILL & SUGARTOWN........................ 218 Bedford Avenue
718-387-7322 bet. N. 4th / N. 5th Streets
STRAND... 828 Broadway
Tel. 212-473-1452 at 12th Street
THREE LIVES & CO... 154 West 10th Street
Tel. 212- 741-2069 at Waverly Place
USED BOOK CAFE...................................... 120 Crosby Street
Tel. 212-334-3324 at Houston Street

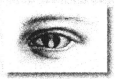
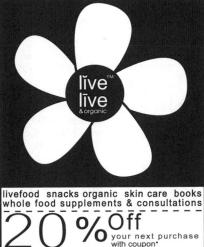
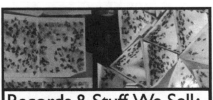

 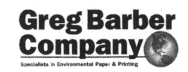

GLOSSARY

Baba ganoush   Middle Eastern spread made of eggplant, tahini, chick peas, lemon garlic.

Bagel   The classic New York bread. Chewy and sprinkled with onion, garlic, or seeds, and shaped like a donut. Eat one and you won't be hungry for hours. Usually vegan; ask about eggs and egg glaze.

Casein   A milk protein that accounts for cheese's ability to melt smoothly. Alas, it is added to nearly all soy cheese, making it unacceptable for vegans.

Chips   To an American, chips are crisps and fries are chips. Get it?

Dim Sum   Asian buffet: a selection of lots of different dumplings, savory cakes and the like.

Eggplant   Aubergine.

Falafel   The vegetarian meatball: a Middle Eastern deep fried patty of ground chick peas, garlic, and parsley.

Gluten   Chewy bland dough made from wheat flour which absorbs the flavors of the dish or sauce it's cooked in, like tofu. Common meat substitute.

Hummus   Middle Eastern spread made of ground chick peas, tahini, garlic, lemon and olive oil.

Knish   A savory pastry in which a simple thin dough is wrapped around a filling of potato, buckwheat, rice, etc. Usually vegan, but it pays to ask about cheese or butter, and whether the dough is made with egg.

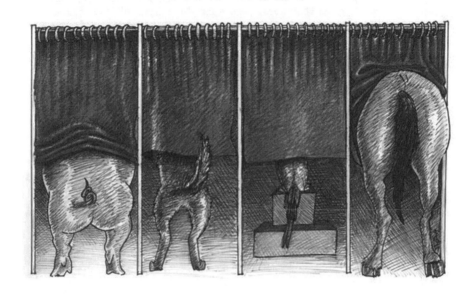

THEY CAN'T VOTE. *YOU CAN.*

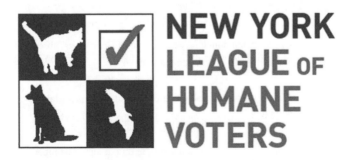

NEW YORK LEAGUE OF HUMANE VOTERS

WWW.NYLHV.ORG

Kosher	Strict dietary guidelines followed by some Jews; they include a prohibition on mixing meat with milk in the same meal or the same kitchen. That means a kosher "dairy" restaurant will have no meat, with lots of options for ovo-lacto vegetarians but nothing for vegans, while a kosher restaurant that serves meat will have no dairy. Likewise, if a processed food is labeled "kosher," it won't contain both animal gelatin and milk powder, for instance.
Macrobiotic	A way of eating from Eastern traditions that seeks to bring foods into balance. Macro restaurants usually serve fish and sometimes eggs, but no dairy; they always have plenty for vegans.
Pico de Gallo	Mexican salsa made from raw onions, tomatoes, garlic, and cilantro.
Pretzel	On the street, these are big warm salty affairs that can stave off hunger in a pinch. They're 100% vegan.
Seitan	Gluten which has been boiled in a gingertamari broth.
Soy cheese	Soy milk processed to approximate the consistency and flavor of cheese. It almost always contains casein, a milk protein, so check to make sure it's vegan. (Soymage and Tofutti are typical brands of vegan cheese.)
Squash	A sweet autumn vegetable that comes in many types; pumpkin is one.
Tempeh	Fermented soybeans pressed into cakes, more flavorful than tofu.
Tempura	Vegetables dipped in batter and deep fried. Ask about eggs in the batter.
Tofu	Tofu is to soy milk as cheese is to cow's milk. Relatively bland, it soaks up the flavors of whatever it's cooked in.
Zucchini	Courgette.

CRUELTY-FREE SHOES

U ntil recently, it was scandalous that in New York, one of the world's great pedestrian cities, there were no shops that specialized in selling vegetarian shoes. But now with the advent of shops like Moo Shoes and 99X, you can buy non-leather shoes that are durable, breathable, and good-looking.

MOOSHOES
78 Orchard Street
bet. Grand/ Broome

Shoes, belts, and wallets all made by companies that make only leather-free goods.
www.mooshoes.com • 212-254-6512

NY ARTIFICIAL

NYA BLUE
13 8th Avenue
at West 12th Street

Shoes, jewelry, accessories, handbags , apparel, and makeup.
www. nyartificial.com • 646-340-0442

PAYLESS SHOE SOURCE
9 NYC locations; check phone book

Inexpensive, leather-look plastic shoes that last about 6 months.

STELLA McCARTNEY
429 West 14th Street

Non-leather shoes, accessories and clothing.
www.stellamccarney.com • 212-255-1556

MARCH 3-4 2012

The Metropolitan Pavilion 125 West 18th Street

www.NYCVegfoodfest.com

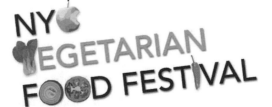

NYC VEGETARIAN FOOD FESTIVAL

WHY VEGANISM?

Vegetarians avoid meat because of the animal suffering, negative health effects, and environmental damage involved in "eating carcasses," as Leo Tolstoy put it. Vegans carry these reasons to their logical conclusion and avoid using all animal products, to the extent possible.

Cruelty

Milk and eggs are taken from animals kept in horrific conditions on factory farms. Hens are packed into cages so small they would peck each other to death if their beaks hadn't been cut off by a hot knife; these cages are jammed into buildings housing as many as 80,000 birds. After a few exhausting years of laying eggs over conveyor belts with fluorescent lights on 18 hours a day, spent hens are turned into soup. In cows, as in women, there is a connection between lactation and pregnancy: cows only give milk after giving birth. Therefore cows are artificially inseminated every year and their calves are taken away to be slaughtered for pet food or raised for veal in confining crates. Cows are injected with hormones to increase their milk output, tranquilizers to calm them down and antibiotics to keep them from succumbing to the diseases they contract from the unhealthy conditions in which they are kept. After five or six years of this treatment they are slaughtered. (The natural lifespan of a cow is 20 years.)

Health

Eggs are high in cholesterol, which contributes to heart disease, the leading killer in the United States. Milk products such as whole milk, cheese and yogurt are high in cholesterol and saturated fat, which has been linked to heart disease and cancer. Even non-fat milk products can be harmful: recent studies have linked milk consumption to cataracts and a diet high in animal protein to osteoporosis; while the Recommended Dietary Allowance of protein (for men) is 63 grams, vegetarian men consume an average of 103 grams. Intolerance of milk is the most common food allergy, leading to flatulence and respiratory and skin problems. The U.S. Department of Agriculture estimates that 50% of the dairy cattle in the herds along Mexico's northern border—whose milk is sold in the U.S.—are infected with tuberculosis. And everything the cow eats, from antibiotics to pesticide-laden grain, winds up in her milk. The American Medical Association states that a vegan diet provides all required nutrients, including calcium, iron, and vitamin B-12. Olympic gold medalist Carl Lewis is a vegan—need we say more?

Environment

Animals are kept in such concentrations in factory farms or feedlots that tons of their wastes, laden with pesticide and chemical residue, become a hazard. Livestock production accounts for a staggering 50 percent of America's fresh water use. The runoff from cleaning stalls is contaminated and pollutes acquifers and rivers. Eighty percent of the herbicides used in the U.S. are sprayed on soybeans and corn, most of which are fed to livestock. Livestock raising is the primary cause of topsoil erosion in the United States, but that doesn't stop the U.S. government from spending $13 billion on price supports for milk. 64 percent of U.S. agricultural land is used for livestock feed. Shouldn't we eat the grain and leave the cow's secretions for her calf?

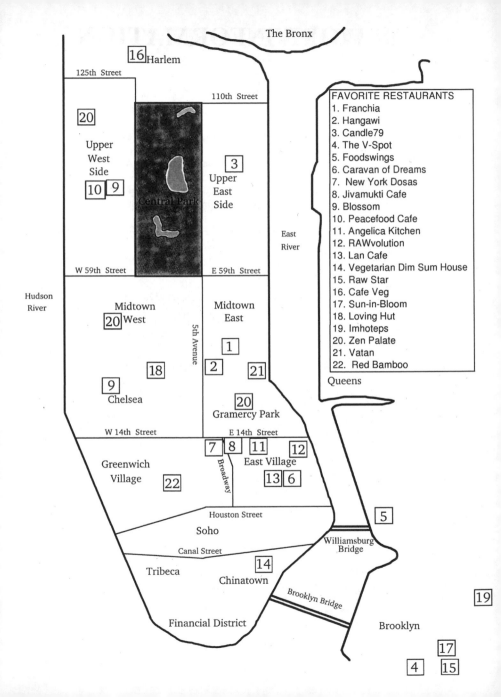

The Bronx

16 Harlem

125th Street

20

Upper West Side

10 9

Central Park

110th Street

3

Upper East Side

East River

FAVORITE RESTAURANTS
1. Franchia
2. Hangawi
3. Candle79
4. The V-Spot
5. Foodswings
6. Caravan of Dreams
7. New York Dosas
8. Jivamukti Cafe
9. Blossom
10. Peacefood Cafe
11. Angelica Kitchen
12. RAWvolution
13. Lan Cafe
14. Vegetarian Dim Sum House
15. Raw Star
16. Cafe Veg
17. Sun-in-Bloom
18. Loving Hut
19. Imhoteps
20. Zen Palate
21. Vatan
22. Red Bamboo

W 59th Street

E 59th Street

Hudson River

Midtown West
20

5th Avenue

Midtown East

1

2

21

18

20

9

Chelsea

Gramercy Park

Queens

W 14th Street

E 14th Street

7 8 11 12

Broadway

East Village

13 6

Greenwich Village

22

Houston Street

Soho

5

Canal Street

Williamsburg Bridge

14

Tribeca

Chinatown

Brooklyn Bridge

19

Financial District

Brooklyn

17

4 15

FOR MORE INFORMATION

ANIMALS, HEALTH, AND THE ENVIRONMENT

Farm Animal Reform Movement,10101 Ashburton Lane, Bethesda, MD 20817; ((888)
FARM-USA: www. FARMUSA.org
Farm Sanctuary-Organization for the Rescue and Protection of Farm Animals,
PO Box 150, Watkins Glen, NY 14891; ☎ (607) 583-2225
United Poultry Concerns, PO Box 150, Machipongo, VA 23405-0150, ☎ (757) 678-7875
Society & Animals Forum, PO Box 1297. Washington Grove, MD. 20880-1297. ☎ (301)
963-4751
Animal People, PO Box 960. Clinton, Washington, 98236-0960, MD. 20880-1297, ☎ (360)
579-2505
People for the Ethical Treatment of Animals, 501 Front Street, Norfolk, VA 23510; ☎ (757)
622-PETA
Friends of Animals 1841 Broadway, #812 , New York, NY 10023, ☎ (212) 247-8120
Animal Legal Defense Fund, 127 Fourth Street, Petaluma, CA 94952, ☎ (707) 769-7771
North American Vegetarian Society, PO Box 72, Dolgeville, NY 13329, ☎ (518)
568-7970
New York League of Humane Voters, 151 First Avenue, Suite 237, New York, NY 10009. ☎/
212-889-0303; www.nylhv.org
American Vegan Society, 56 Dinshah Lane, PO Box 360, Malaga, NJ 08328, ☎ (856)
694-2887
Institute for Integrative Nutrition, 3 East 28th Street, 12th floor, NYC, NY 10016☎ (212)
730-5433. Offers natural cooking classes with no animal products.
Institute for Food and Health and The Natural Gourmet School, 48 West 21st St., 2nd Floor,
☎ (212) 645-5170. Natural cooking classes and a $20 Friday night vegan feast.
Earth Save New York, PO Box 96, NY, NY 10108, ☎ (212) 696-7986

VEGAN DELIGHTS

Vegan Catering in NYC: www. Ecocheflove.com; Chef@mamaearthrocks.com ☎(877) 833-
1336
Vegan Chocolate Decadence, ☎ (800) 324-5018
Vegan Dried Fruits-Rainforest Delights, ☎ (626) 284-8001
Vegan Parmesan, Parma, ☎ (541) 665-0346
Vegan Organic Produce Home Delivery Service-Urban Organic, ☎ (415) 412-1336
Vegan Organic Cookies and Brownies-Allison's Gourmet, ☎ (800) 361-8292

✉ FEEDBACK ✉

Please write to let us know how we can improve the next edition of The Vegan Guide to New York City. Tell us about new restaurants, changes, closings, great meals, whatever you like.

_____
_____
_____
_____
_____
Your address: _____
_____
_
_____
_____

Additional copies.

For additional copies of The Vegan Guide to New York City, send $9.95 plus $3.00 postage each to:

Rynn Berry, 159 Eastern Parkway,
Suite 2H, Brooklyn, NY 11238.
tele/fax: (718) 622-8002.
Email: berrynn@att.net.
Web: vegsource.com/berry.
www. veganguidetonyc.com

ALSO AVAILABLE: Rynn Berry's other bestselling books:
• *Famous Vegetarians* and *Their Favorite Recipes* @ $16.95 plus $3.00 postage.
• *Food for the Gods: Vegetarianism and the World's Religions* @ $19.95 plus $3.00 postage.
• *Hitler: Neither Vegetarian Nor Animal Lover* @ $10.95 plus $3.00 postage.
•*The New Vegetarians* @ $10.95 plus $3.00 postage
• *Becoming Raw* @ $24.95 plus $3.00 postage.
For copies of:
The Vegan Passport @ $5.00;Vegetarian London @ $10.00;
Vegetarian Britain @ $13.50; Vegetarian France @ $12.00;
Vegetarian Europe @ $13.50; send the designated amount, plus $3.00 postage, to Attention: Freya Dinshah, The American Vegan Society, 56 Dinshah Lane, PO Box 360, Malaga, NJ 08328 USA.

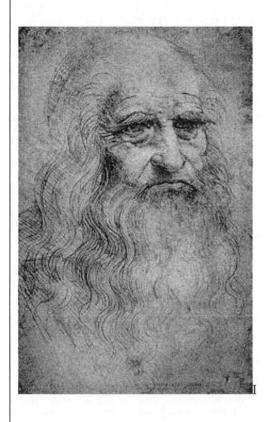

I have from an early age abjured the use of meat, and the time will come when men such as I will look upon the murder of animals as they now look upon the murder of men.

LEONARDO DA VINCI, 1452-1519
Artist, scientist, inventor, engineer, architect
"Renaissance Man"

Best Vegan Bites-2012

Best Appetizer: Jalapeno Hush Puppies @ Dirt Candy; The Hawaiian Roll @ Nature & Organic Life Café (in Flushing, Queens).

Best Salad: The Other Caesar @ Peacefood Café/Angel's Salad @ Caravan of Dreams.

Best Soup: The Pho @ Lan Café; Udon Noodle Soup @ Loving Hut.

Best Veggie Burger: The Big Matt "Cheese" Burger @ RAWvolution.

Best Sandwiches: Pan-Seared French Horn Mushrooms Panini @ Peacefood Café/ Vegan BLT @ The V-Spot: The Midtown Melt @ Blossom du Jour.

Best Smoothie: Rain Forest Smoothie @ The Juice Press.

Best Entrée: Tofu and Roasted Kabocha Pumpkin in Sesame Soy Sauce @ Franchia/ Seitan Piccata @ Candle 79; Wild Rice & Cremini Risotto Croquettes @ Caravan of Dreams.,

Best Rice Dish: Bibenbap @ Franchia; Pineapple Fried Rice @ Wild Ginger

Best Noodles: Kim Chee Noodles, and Jap Chae Noodles @ Wild Ginger (Smith Street}; Spaghetti Bolognese @ The V-Note.

Best Pizza: Mushroom Quxelle@ Peacefood Café.

Best Wrap: The Tempeh Wrap @ FoodSwings.

Best French Fries: French Fries @ FoodSwings.

Best Pastry: The Triple-Berry Danish and the Cinnamon Swirls @ Champs Bakery (Williamsburg, Brooklyn).

Best Dessert: Wheat Free Chocolate Mousse Pie @ Candle Café.

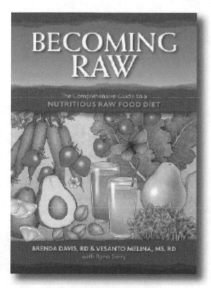

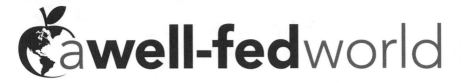
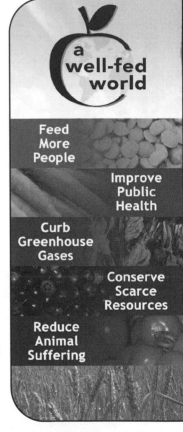
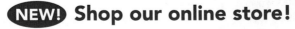